Physiological Society Study Guides   *Number 4*

Neuronal communications

Physiological Society Study Guides

Physiological Society Study Guides   *Number 4*

Neuronal communications

Edited by
W. Winlow

Manchester University Press

Manchester and New York

Distributed exclusively in the USA and Canada by St. Martin's Press

Published by Manchester University Press
Oxford Road, Manchester M13 9PL, UK
and Room 400, 175 Fifth Avenue,
New York, NY 10010, USA

*Distributed exclusively in the USA and Canada
by* St. Martin's Press, Inc.,
175 Fifth Avenue, New York, NY 10010, USA

British Library cataloguing in publication data
Neuronal communications.
1. Animals. Neurons. Biochemistry
I. V''nlow, W. (William)
591.1'88

Library of Congress cataloguing in publication data
Neuronal communications / edited by W. Winlow.
  p. cm.
  Bibliography: p.
  ISBN 0-7190-2828-0.—ISBN 0-7190-2829-9 (pbk.)
  1. Synapses. 2. Neurotransmitters. 3. Neurotransmitter
receptors. 4. Neurons. I. Winlow, W. (William)
  [DNLM: 1. Neural Transmission. 2. Neurons—physiology.
3. Neuroregulators. 4. Synapses—physiology. WL 102.5 N49355]
QP364.N45   1989
599'.0188—dc20
DNLM/DLC
for Library of Congress   89-12770

ISBN 0 7190 2828 0 *hardback*
ISBN 0 7190 2829 9 *paperback*

Typeset in Hong Kong
by Graphicraft Typesetters Ltd., Hong Kong

Printed in Great Britain
by Biddles Ltd., Guildford and King's Lynn

Contents

Contributors

G. J. Dockray Physiological Laboratory, University of Liverpool, Brownlow Hill, P.O. Box 147, Liverpool L69 3BX

H. Ghazi Nuffield Laboratory of Ophthalmology, Walton Street, Oxford OX2 6AW

W. J. Heitler The Gatty Marine Laboratory, University of St Andrews, St Andrews, Fife KY16 8LB

D. J. Maxwell Department of Preclinical Veterinary Sciences, University of Edinburgh, Summerhall, Edinburgh EH9 1QH

N. N. Osborne Nuffield Laboratory of Ophthalmology, Walton Street, Oxford OX2 6AW

P. J. Simmons Department of Zoology, University of Newcastle upon Tyne, Newcastle upon Tyne NE1 7RU

A. B. Tobin Nuffield Laboratory of Ophthalmology, Walton Street, Oxford OX2 6AW

W. Winlow Department of Physiology, The Worsley Medical and Dental Building, University of Leeds, Leeds LS2 9NQ

Prologue
The 'typical' neurone

W. Winlow Department of Physiology, University of Leeds

> People know about quite different things, and this often makes conversation difficult. Rose Macaulay, *The Towers of Trebizond*, 1956, p. 42 (Collins, London).

It has always been very clear to neuroscientists that there is no such thing as a typical neurone, but many of us when faced with students *en masse* have used the alpha motoneurone as a typical example of what a nerve cell should look like. Nothing really could be further from the truth (as is demonstrated by David Maxwell in Chapter 1), but alpha motoneurones have features which tempt us to use them as a teaching aid for physiologists and anatomists alike. In Figure 0.1 they are shown to have dendrites and a cell body which receive synaptic inputs and which conduct decrementally, and axons which conduct regeneratively and are the sole outputs from the cell, via the axon terminals (through which transmitter release across the cell membrane takes place – see Chapter 3).

Perhaps it is better for us to consider that neurones are really stretched secretory cells, sometimes connected to one another by electrical synapses which, in the case of the alpha motoneurone, are specialised to signal over long distances (tens of centimetres) at speed. The discovery of the nature of that signal, the action potential, was of critical importance to our understanding of modern neurophysiology, but action potentials are basically a mechanism for switching on a secretory process at a distance from a cell body and many short neurones, in both vertebrates and invertebrates, do not have the ability to discharge action potentials. This is shown by Peter Simmons in Chapter 4.

It is perhaps ironic that the great controversy between those

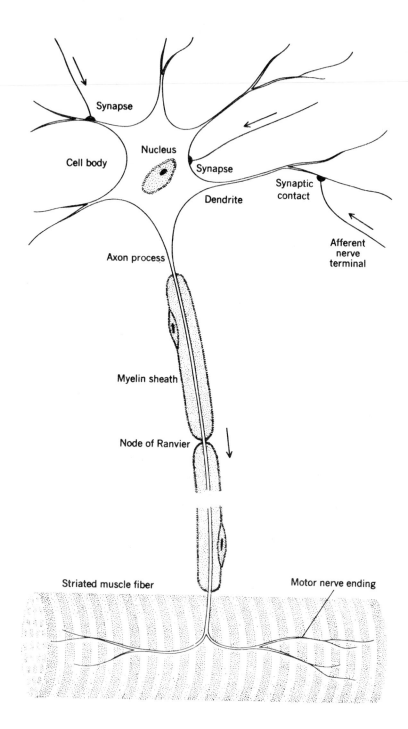

Synapse

Nucleus

Cell body

Synapse

Synaptic
contact

Dendrite

Afferent
nerve
terminal

Axon process

Myelin sheath

Node of Ranvier

Striated muscle fiber

Motor nerve ending

who believed that synaptic transmission was by chemical means and those who believed that the nervous system was a functional syncytium in which all cells were in electrical continuity with one another, when finally resolved in the late 1950s, showed that both parties were right! Both electrical and chemical synapses exist, so that although neurones may be considered as single entities within the nervous system, many are indeed part of a functional syncytium. Bill Heitler demonstrates, in Chapter 2, that electrical synapses may be complex and have integrative capabilities which are not widely understood.

Back at the beginning of the evolution of the Metazoa, it is probable that small, soft-bodied animals did not possess neurones with action potentials, but the secretory process was of prime importance. For many years we laboured under the delusion that only a very small number of neurotransmitters existed, but over recent years many more have been discovered, particularly the peptide neurotransmitters and neuromodulators which Graham Dockray considers in Chapter 5. In addition, the mistaken view was taken that only a single transmitter substance would emanate from any given nerve terminal, but this view largely collapsed in the late 1970s. This is discussed by Andrew Tobin and Neville Osborne in Chapter 6. However, the phenomenon of physiological 'co-transmission' is still to be confirmed. Finally, the role of glial tissue is now emerging as one of fundamental importance to

---

Fig. 0.1 An 'orthodox' neurone (spinal motoneurone of frog), showing its incoming central synaptic inputs and its peripheral output at a neuro-muscular junction. In neurones of this type, the dendrites receive synaptic inputs, integrate them and conduct them decrementally towards the cell body, where further synaptic inputs are received and further integration takes place. A spike (action potential) generator resides at the base of the axon process (usually termed the axon hillock) and action potentials are conducted regeneratively from here to the motor nerve-endings, where transmitter is released onto the postjunctional folds of the muscle after the spike has invaded the presynaptic terminal. Whilst this is an excellent model for teaching purposes, the majority of central neurones do not have this type of structure and many lack action potentials, which should not be considered a diagnostic feature of neurones. (From Katz 1966.)

neural tissue. This is discussed in detail in Chapter 7 by Ghazi and Osborne. Thus neurones, and their investing glia, may have many forms and variable functional characteristics. None can be said to be typical or to be specific diagnostic features. In this collection of chapters I have tried to draw together modern views on how nerve cells signal to one another and to set them into the context of previous knowledge.

Reference

Katz, B. (1966). *Nerve Muscle and Synapse*. McGraw-Hill, New York.

1

Modern techniques for investigating the structure of neurones

D. J. Maxwell Department of Preclinical Veterinary Sciences, University of Edinburgh

1.1 Introduction

Over the past decade or so there has been a resurgence of interest in neuroanatomy. This has arisen principally as a result of the development of a large number of new anatomical techniques. These techniques provide analytical tools of great potency which enable us to ask questions of the nervous system which would previously have been difficult, or even impossible, to answer. It is not the purpose of this article to supply step-by-step instructions in the various techniques but rather to inform the reader of what can be achieved using them.

In a short-chapter it is not feasible to cover all neuroanatomical techniques; also, new approaches are developing so rapidly that omissions are inevitable. What follows is an account of various modern techniques which have significantly advanced our understanding of the mammalian nervous system in recent years. Initially I shall consider the aims of modern neuroanatomical studies. The techniques themselves will be discussed under four headings:

Tract-tracing methods
Intracellular staining
Immunocytochemistry
Golgi methods.

Finally, exciting advances achieved by combining different techniques will also be described.

1.2 Aims of anatomical studies

The general aim of neuroanatomical studies is to determine the organisation of the nervous system in the hope that such knowledge will improve our understanding of how it functions. The types of question asked may be arbitrarily divided into three classes:

(i) Questions which are concerned with *location*: for example, we may wish to locate the cells of origin of a pathway or a peripheral nerve or to determine the projections of axons originating from a nucleus. This type of problem is usually tackled using one of the tract-tracing methods. Alternatively if the aim of the study is to map the distribution of neurones with similar chemical composition or of certain physiological characteristics it will be necessary to use immunocytochemistry or intracellular staining respectively.

(ii) Questions about *arborisation patterns*: we may wish to know if the dendritic or axonal arbor of a particular type of neurone is confined to certain regions of the neuropil or if the arbor is orientated in a particular way. Details of branching patterns and numbers of branch points formed by dendritic arbors may also be useful or constructing and testing biophysical models of neurones. Intracellular staining and the Golgi technique are most useful for providing this sort of data.

(iii) Questions concerning *synaptic organisation*: for example, knowledge of the synaptic arrangements formed by an axon terminal can reveal how it influences its postsynaptic targets. Most questions of this type can only be answered by examining neurones or their axons with the electron microscope. Many anatomical techniques can now be combined with electron microscopy and this approach has enabled researchers to determine synaptic arrangements formed by specific types of neurones or axons which have been characterised using one of the techniques. We may also wish to know about synaptic connections between individual neurones or groups of neurones; the combination of various anatomical techniques has enabled direct observations to be made of the synaptic relationships formed between neurones and has greatly increased our understanding of neuronal networks.

Many of the techniques to be discussed can be used to answer more than one of the three types of question and some of them provide additional information; for example, intracellular staining provides electrophysiological data and immunocytochemistry reveals the chemical composition of neurones.

1.3 Tract-tracing methods

Tract-tracing methods employ substances which are readily taken up by axon terminals or somata of neurones but not by axons of passage. Once a tracer substance has been taken up it is transported along the axon to other regions of the neurone and its presence can be identified by a variety of means. These methods tend to be less capricious and provide more detail than traditional approaches based on degeneration (e.g. see Walberg, 1964) and have provided much new information about efferent and afferent projections of the nervous system. The book by Heimer & Robards (1981) provides an excellent overview of tract-tracing. Four classes of tracer will be considered in this section:

Horseradish peroxidase
Lectins and toxins
Fluorescent substances
Radioactive tracers.

1.3.1 *Horseradish peroxidase*
As its name implies horseradish peroxidase (HRP) is an enzyme extracted from the root of the horseradish. HRP readily forms a complex with hydrogen peroxide (its substrate) which oxidises compounds known as chromogens. In their oxidised state, chromogens precipitate to form a visible reaction product. HRP is taken up by neurones by a process of endocytosis and transported in both the anterograde and retrograde directions (see Mesulam, 1982, for a review). Thus, its presence in neurones can be revealed histochemically by expoiting the oxidative reaction. A number of different chromogens have been used including DAB (3,3′-diaminobenzidine tetrahydrochloride) (Graham &

Karnowsky, 1966), PCPD (pyrocatechol/p-phenylenediamine) (Hanker *et al.*, 1977) and TMB (3,3′,5,5′-tetramethylbenzidine) (Mesulam, 1978). All of these chromogens form electron-dense reaction products and therefore can be used in combination with electron microscopical techniques. The TMB method is the most sensitive but forms a crystalline reaction product which can obscure detail, especially at the ultrastructural level. HRP has been used extensively to label neurones by retrograde transport (Figure 1.1A and B). The earliest demonstrations of retrograde transport of HRP were by Kristensson & Olsson (1971), who injected a solution of HRP into a muscle and were able to trace the motor neurones innervating the muscle in the spinal cord; La Vail & La Vail (1972) used retrograde transport of HRP to trace visual pathways in the central nervous system of the chick. Since these two pioneering studies there have been numerous reports showing that HRP is useful for identifying cells of origin of peripheral nerves and central pathways. Ultrastructural studies of retrogradely labelled neurones (e.g. La Vail & La Vail, 1974) show that reaction product is incorporated into membrane-bound structures or multivesicular bodies (Figure 1.1C). It is therefore possible to identify retrogradely labelled cells with the electron microscope and to examine synaptic boutons in contact with them. Anterograde tracing with HRP has not been used as extensively as retrograde labelling but if sensitive chromogens and/or electron microscopy are employed, axon terminals of neurones that have taken up exogenous HRP can be identified (Lynch *et al.*, 1973; Brownson *et al.*, 1977; Mesulam & Mufson, 1980; Schönitzer & Holländer, 1981).

Another approach to tracing neuronal connections with HRP has been to use the 'injury filling' phenomenon. If a nerve or tract is deliberately severed and HRP is placed on the lesion, either in solution or as a solid pellet, it is possible to label axonal projections (Proshansky & Egger, 1977) and/or cells of origin (Oldfield & McLachlan, 1977; Enevoldson *et al.* 1984). Axons, isolated from their parent cells, are only labelled for a few millimetres and movement of HRP appears to be by passive diffusion. Conversely, retrograde labelling from severed axons occurs over considerable distances and the label is actively transported. Ultrastructural properties of primary afferent terminals in the

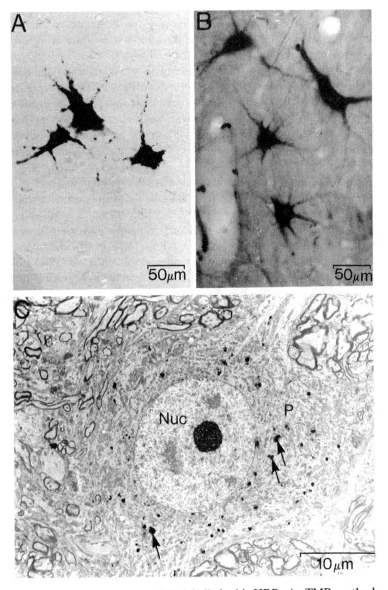

Fig. 1.1 Neurones retrogradely labelled with HRP: A, TMB method;
B, PCPD method; C, electron micrograph of neurone labelled with the
PCPD method. Note the dense membrane-bound bodies containing
reaction product (arrows). (Nuc. = nucleus, P = perikaryon.)

spinal cord labelled by injury filling have been described by Beattie *et al.* (1978). In this case the reaction product is diffuse and not packaged into organelles. HRP has been used to map the central terminations of sensory nerves innervating various peripheral organs. The enzyme is either injected into the organ or placed on a severed distal branch of the nerve innervating the organ and is transported across dorsal root ganglia to the central branches of the spinal nerves and labels their central terminations (Grant *et al.*, 1979; Mesulam & Brushart, 1979). HRP has proved to be a versatile tracer and has few disadvantages. The greatest problem with HRP is that injection sites tend to be large and messy and are difficult to confine to discrete regions of the nervous system. Furthermore, dendritic trees of neurones are only partially labelled and HRP is of limited use for tracing axonal projections. Further applications of HRP, in conjunction with lectins and toxins, intracellular staining and immunohistochemistry are discussed below.

1.3.2 *Lectins and toxins*
Lectins and toxins bind with high affinity to membrane-bound glycocoproteins and glycolipids and are incorporated into neurones by a process of adsorptive endocytosis (for reviews see Trojanowski, 1983; Sawchenko & Gerfen, 1985). It has been estimated that conjugates of wheat-germ agglutinin (WGA) and cholera toxin (CT) are 30–50 times more sensitive than free HRP which is taken up by neurones by bulk endocytosis (Trojanowski *et al.*, 1981). They therefore can be injected in small quantities and avoid the problem of large injection sites encountered with HRP.

WGA has been used extensively in the peripheral and central nervous system as a retrograde, anterograde and transganglionic tracer and it is generally agreed that it is more potent than HRP. The presence of WGA in neurones can be demonstrated autoradiographically (Schwab *et al.*, 1978) or immunocytochemically (Ruda & Coulter, 1982), but it is most commonly conjugated to HRP (Gonatas *et al.*, 1979) and revealed by standard HRP histochemistry. HRP-conjugated WGA therefore can be used in conjunction with electron microscopy and is particularly useful for anterograde tracing of axon terminals (e.g. Flink & Westman, 1985). One further advantage of WGA (and also a potential disadvantage) is that it is transneuronally transported both anterogradely (Gerfen *et al.*, 1982; Itaya & van Hoesen, 1982; Ruda & Coulter; 1982) and retrogradely (Harrison *et al.*, 1984) and thus can be used to trace chains of neurones.

CT shares many of the advantages of WGA over HRP and has been used in the peripheral nervous system as a retrograde and anterograde tracer (Trojanowski *et al.*, 1981) and, like WGA, it is transneuronally transported (Trojanowski & Schmidt, 1984). CT is particularly useful for revealing details of dendritic arbors of retrogradely labelled neurones (Wan *et al.*, 1982). Tetanus toxin has also been employed to trace neuronal pathways and is transneuronally transported (Schwab & Thoenen, 1976).

It is usually not possible to resolve individual axon fibres and details of terminals with HRP, WGA and CT anterograde tracing techniques at the light microscopical level. However, recently a lectin, *Phaseolus vulgaris*-leucoagglutinin (PHA-L), which is extracted from the red kidney bean has been employed as a specific anterograde tracer (Gerfen & Sawchenko, 1984; Groenwegen & van Dijk, 1984). PHA-L is ionophoresed in minute quantities into the central nervous system and is taken up by neurones and transported in the anterograde direction. The presence of PHA-L in neurones is revealed by immunochemical techniques. Neurones at the injection site are well-labelled and have a Golgi-like appearance but the principal advantage of this technique is that individual axon fibres and their terminal specialisations can be clearly resolved (Figure 1.2A). Neurones and axon terminals labelled with PHA-L can be examined with the electron microscope (Wouterlood & Gronwegen, 1985) in order to assess the synaptic arrangements that they form (Figure 1.2B).

1.3.3 *Fluorescent substances*
A number of fluorescent substances including Evans blue, Primuline, bisbenzamide and propidium iodide have proved to be useful retrograde tracers of neurones (Kuypers *et al.*, 1977; 1979). Some substances such as bisbenzamide and Nuclear Yellow selectively label nuclei whereas others such as True or Fast Blue label the cytoplasm (Bentivoglio *et al.*, 1980b; Kuypers *et al.*, 1980).

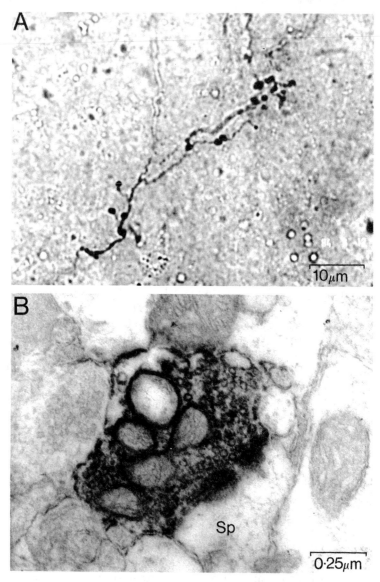

Fig. 1.2 A, Axon terminals in the rat's cortex labelled with PHA-L.
(micrograph by courtesy of G. W. Arbuthnot). B, An electron micrograph of a PHA-L labelled bouton: Sp = a dendritic spine postsynaptic to the labelled bouton.

Fluorescent dyes are especially useful for double-labelling experiments where two tracers are required to demonstrate neurones with divergent collateral projections (van der Kooy *et al.*, 1978; Kuypers *et al.*, 1980). Different tracers may be identified in the same neurone by differences in their excitation wavelengths or their ability selectively to label different regions of a cell. These techniques are advantageous in that they are fast and easy to use; however, labelled neurones tend to fade after some time and some tracers can diffuse out of neurones and label surrounding glial cells (Bentivoglio *et al.*, 1980a).

1.3.4 Radioactive tracers

Radioactivity can be identified in tissue by autoradiographic techniques (see Rogers, 1979, for a review). Axonal projections of neurones have been extensively studied with tritiated amino acids which are taken up by somata, incorporated into proteins and transported down the axon in the anterograde direction (Droz & Le Blond, 1963; Goldberg & Kontani, 1967; Cowan *et al.*, 1972). Some radioactive tracers such as proline are transported transneuronally and have been particularly useful for tracing pathways in the visual system (Grafstein, 1971; Wiesel *et al.*, 1974). Autoradiographic techniques can be extended to the ultrastructural level; therefore it is possible to examine the synaptic arrangements formed by labelled axon terminals (e.g. Hendrickson, 1972; Le Vay and Gilbert, 1976).

Injection sites of radioisotopes are diffuse and difficult to define and it can be difficult to determine the terminal region of a labelled pathway. Autoradiography is also time-consuming, particularly at the electron microscopical level.

Autoradiography is also of use in assessing metabolic activity in neurones (Korr, 1981). In particular, the 2-deoxyglucose technique (Sokoloff *et al.*, 1977) can demonstrate activity in neuronal systems in response to applied or natural stimuli.

A further application of radioactive tracing is the identification of neurones that selectively take up labelled transmitter substances or their precursors (e.g. Streit *et al.*, 1978; Streit, 1980).

1.4 Intracellular staining techniques

Intracellular staining techniques employ recording micropipettes containing marker substances such as HRP, cobalt chloride or Lucifer yellow. Neurones or their axons are impaled and identified by electrophysiological criteria prior to introducing marker substances into them by pressure injection or microionophoresis. Suitable markers must be retained within neurones and must not diffuse out through membranes. These techniques have two considerable advantages over Golgi and other methods for revealing the structures of neurones:

(i) They produce electrophysiological and morphological data and thus provide a unique opportunity to correlate structural and functional properties of neurones.

(ii) Single neurones or their axons are impaled and therefore individual labelled structures can be identified with confidence in sections or wholemount preparations.

Overviews of intracellular staining techniques are provided in the books by Kater & Nicholson (1973) and Brown & Fyffe (1984), and the review by Bishop & King (1982).

Stretton & Kravitz (1968) were the first to demonstrate intracellular staining of neurones in the abdominal ganglion of the lobster using the fluorescent dye Procion Yellow. Subsequently the Procion Yellow technique was also successfully applied to the mammalian central nervous system; e.g. Jankowska & Lindström (1970). However it soon became apparent that Procion Yellow did not reveal the finest details of dendrites and axons and therefore provided only a limited picture of neuronal geometry. Furthermore the dye contained no heavy atom and therefore could only be used indirectly in conjunction with electron microscopy (Purves & McMahan, 1972). Another fluorescent dye, Lucifer Yellow, was introduced by Stewart (1978, 1981) as an intracellular marker. Unlike Procion, Lucifer Yellow completely fills the finest processes of neurones and is useful for revealing dendrites, spines, axons and axon collaterals. Lucifer Yellow can be visualised in living neurones and, as no histochemical processing is required, it may satisfactorily be used in wholemount preparations and in slices of nervous tissue. Lucifer Yellow itself is not electron-dense but neurones labelled with it may be rendered electron-opaque by exposing them to a photo-oxidation reaction in the presence of diaminobenzidine (Maranto, 1982). Finally, both Procion and Lucifer Yellow pass readily through gap junctions (with the exception of those of gastropod molluscs) and therefore may be used to demonstrate electrical coupling between neurones (Payton *et al.*, 1969; Stewart, 1978). Cobalt chloride is an intracellular marker that has been chiefly applied to invertebrate or amphibian preparations (Pitman *et al.*, 1972; Gillette & Pomeranz, 1973). Detailed neuronal labelling is revealed when tissue is treated with ammonium sulphide or diaminobenzidine. However, cobalt is toxic to neurones and can alter their physiological characteristics and also blocks microelectrodes (Tweedle, 1978). Therefore valuable physiological data tends to be lost. Ultrastructural preservation of tissue is also usually poor.

The intracellular staining and recording technique with HRP was simultaneously developed in the mid 1970s by a number of groups (Cullheim & Kellereth, 1976; Jankowska *et al.*, 1976; Kitai *et al.*, 1976; Light & Durcovic, 1976; Muller & McMahan 1976; Snow *et al.*, 1976) and has become the technique of choice for investigating neurones of the mammalian central nervous system. HRP has many advantages over the other markers: It is non-toxic and recordings can be made from impaled neurones before and after introducing it. It labels neurones with a Golgi-like fill and even myelinated axons may be traced for a centimetre or more. In addition, HRP reaction product is electron-dense and it is possible to achieve good ultrastructural preservation of processed tissue.

Microelectrodes containing HRP can be used to impale cells (Figure 1.3A) and axons to reveal their structures (e.g. see Brown, 1981). As reagents used to demonstrate HRP activity do not penetrate tissue through great distances it is usual to section blocks prior to performing the reaction. This necessitates reconstruction of the labelled structure from serial sections. Reconstructions are usually made with the help of a drawing tube attachment on the microscope but more recently computer-aided image analysis techniques have been developed for reconstruction (e.g. Houchin *et al.*, 1983; Heitler, 1984).

As an electron-opaque reaction product is produced with HRP the technique can be readily applied to ultrastructural studies (Figure 1.3B) (Cullheim & Kellereth, 1976; Jankowska *et al.*, 1976). Combined light and electron microscopical studies of neurones are performed on sections flat-embedded in resin (e.g. see Metz *et al.*, 1982; Maxwell *et al.*, 1984a). Initially structures are photographed and and reconstructed under the light microscope and areas of interest are selected for ultrastructural analysis; this is achieved by attaching the area to a block and sectioning it on an ultramicrotome. Thin sections are collected on grids and examined with the electron microscope. Thus it is possible to identify the same structures under the light and electron microscope. This approach offers distinct advantages over traditional methods for analysing the neuropil. Firstly it facilitates the identification of structures within the neuropil. Secondly it allows us to verify that structures observed at the light microscopic level are genuine and not artefactual. Finally, it enables direct correlations between the ultrastructure and physiology of neurones to be made.

HRP has few disadvantages as an intracellular marker; a drawback is that it is only possible to trace axons over a centimetre or so before they fade. Also it may be difficult to impale very small structures. Recently Suguria *et al.* (1986) have traced unmyelinated afferent axons in the spinal cord by impaling their dorsal-root ganglion cells with microelectrodes containing PHA-L which is transported for considerable distances.

1.5 Immunocytochemical techniques

There is a variety of immunocytochemical techniques but they all depend upon the ability of antibodies to bind to specific substances (antigens). Antibodies are serum proteins (immunoglobulins) and are produced by immunising an animal against the appropriate antigen, either in pure form or coupled to a larger molecule (e.g. see Forssmann *et al.*, 1981). Specific antibodies are extracted from crude antiserum by means of affinity chromatography. Antibodies produced by this method are heterologous; however, it is also possible to produce identical highly specific monoclonal antibodies by hybrid myeloma technology (Köhler &

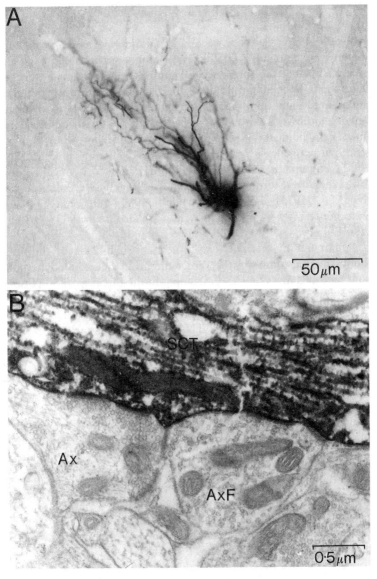

Fig. 1.3 A, A spinocervical tract neurone that was intracellularly labelled with HRP (micrograph by courtesy of Professor A. G. Brown). B,
An electron micrograph of an HRP-labelled dendrite of a spinocervical
tract (SCT) cell: Ax and AxF are boutons presynaptic to the labelled
structure.

Milstein, 1975; Cuello *et al.*, 1980). Immunocytochemical techniques have been particularly useful to neuroscientists for demonstrating the presence of putative neurotransmitters in neurones. Specific antibodies are available for most peptide, monoamine and amino-acid transmitters or enzymes involved in their synthesis. However it should not be forgotten that immunocytochemistry is also useful for identifying other components of neurones (e.g. see Barnstable, 1980; Zipster & McKay, 1981; Triller *et al.*, 1985). Books on immunocytochemical techniques include: Sternberger (1979), Cuello, (1983), Polak & van Noorden (1973), Polak & Varndell (1984) and Childs (1986). Excellent reviews have been writen by De Mey (1983) and van den Pol (1984).

A number of methods exist for the visualisation of the antibody-antigen complex: the direct method; the indirect method; and methods involving several steps. In the direct method (Coons & Kaplan, 1950) a suitable marker such as fluorescein isothiocyanate (FITC), HRP, ferritin or colloidal gold is conjugated to a specific antibody. This method is relatively insensitive and there is the additional difficulty of obtaining specific antibodies conjugated to suitable markers. The indirect method (Avrameas, 1969) employs a specific primary antibody and a labelled second antibody which was raised against immunoglobulins of the species providing the primary antiserum (i.e. an antibody to the primary antibody). The sensitivity of this method is greater than the direct method and second antibodies conjugated to suitable markers are readily available. The peroxidase-antiperoxidase (PAP) method of Sternberger *et al.* (1970) is by far the most popular technique for revealing antibody–antigen complexes. A specific primary antibody is used which is followed by an unlabelled second antibody and finally by a PAP complex which has been raised in the same species as the primary antibody. The PAP complex binds to the second antibody which forms a bridge between it and the primary antibody–antigen complex. The presence of peroxidase is then revealed using standard HRP histochemistry. The PAP method is extremely sensitive and can be used with low dilutions of primary antiserum. A technique that is said to be even more sensitive than PAP has been introduced by Hsu *et al.* (1981) This is the avidin–biotin–peroxidase complex (ABC) method and utilises a biotinylated second antibody followed by the ABC complex. Biotin has a high affinity to avidin and binds to free sites in the ABC complex. It is also possible to bind avidin to other probes such as gold or Texas Red. Finally, protein A which is extracted from the cell wall of *Staphylococcus aureus* binds to some mammalian immunoglobulin molecules and, as colloidal gold can be adsorbed to it, is a useful marker (Roth, 1982).

The choice of method and marker employed depends upon the type of study to be undertaken and also to some extent on the antigen to be exposed. Fluorescent probes are useful for light microscopic studies on frozen and paraffin-embedded sections but fluorescence tends to fade after some time and also it is not possible to view labelled and unlabelled structures simultaneously. Techniques employing peroxidase markers, such as the PAP and ABC techniques, are suitable for light and electron microscopical studies (Figure 1.4) and it is usual to perform correlated light and electron microscopical studies on flat-embedded Vibratome sections.

Ultrastructural studies employing PAP and ABC pre-embedding techniques have their limitations. Firstly, in order to retain antigenicity, it may be necessary to reduce the concentration of glutaraldehyde in fixative solutions; this will inevitably lead to a reduction in the quality of ultrastructural preservation. Secondly, use of detergents or freeze–thawing, which facilitate penetration of antibodies, damage ultrastructure and therefore are usually omitted in ultrastructural studies; this limits penetration to a few microns from the surface of the section. Finally, the reaction product is diffuse and is found throughout the cytoplasm of a labelled cell or axon terminal; therefore it is not possible to identify neuronal compartments such as vesicles that contain antigen. Post-embedding labelling techniques using colloidal gold probes can overcome many of these problems (e.g. see van den Pol, 1984). Staining is performed directly on thin sections mounted on gold or nickel grids and under the electron microscope gold particles are seen to label specific structures, e.g. dense-core vesicles in visceral nerves (Probert *et al.*, 1981; Wharton *et al.*, 1981). By using antibodies raised in different species and gold particles of different diameter it is possible to differentiate between two antigens in the same tissue.

Immunocytochemical techniques have numerous applications

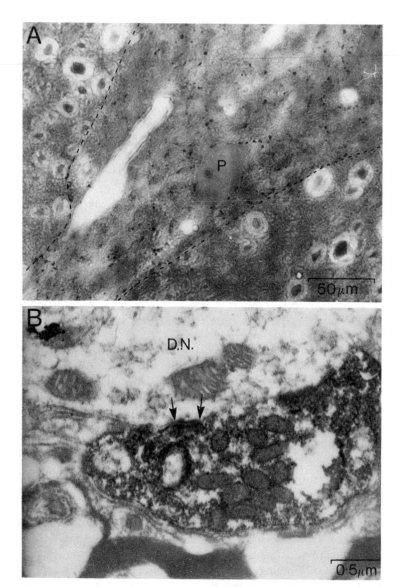

Fig. 1.4 A, Glutamic acid decarboxylase-immunoreactive axons in the lateral cervical nucleus (demarcated by dotted line) of the cat. Note the accumulation of terminals around a neurone (P). (ABC pre-embedding method; plastic embedded section.) B, An electron micrograph of a glutamic acid decarboxylase bouton that is presynaptic to a giant Deiters' neurone (D.N.) in the lateral vestibular nucleus. (ABC pre-embedding method; arrows indicate synapse).

in neuroscience. Individually they can be used to demonstrate the presence of various putative neurotransmitters or other substances in neurones and/or axon terminals. In combination it is possible to demonstrate the coexistence of two or more substances in the same neurone or the relationships between neurones containing different antigens. One golden rule of immunocytochemistry is that it is always necessary to perform careful controls with each experiment.

1.6 Golgi methods

The Golgi method was developed in the last century (Golgi, 1873) and was perfected by Cajal (1909). The reader may be surprised to find it included in a review of modern anatomical techniques but it is still useful for revealing details of neuronal geometry, especially when intracellular staining is not available or difficult to perform, e.g. to examine arborisation patterns of small cells (Maxwell, 1985) or neurones with short axons (Somogyi, 1978). Furthermore, it is feasible to combine the technique with electron microscopy (Blackstad, 1970, 1981) and therefore synaptic relationships of impregnated neurones can be assessed.

The black precipitate formed in neurones during the Golgi procedure is silver chromate. Neurones impregnated with silver chromate can be examined in thin sections under the electron microscope (e.g. Somogyi, 1978). However the precipitate is dense and masks details of labelled elements and also is soluble in water and dissolves during collection and staining of sections. In order to overcome these difficulties Fairén *et al.* (1977) developed the 'Gold Toning' method of substituting particles of metallic gold for silver chromate (Figure 1.5). As the gold is particulate, it does not obscure intracellular details nor dissolve in water.

The Golgi method is notoriously capricious; often several attempts are necessary to stain the required class of neurone. Also it is difficult to maintain good ultrastructural preservation in tissue prepared for combined light and electron microscopy. Finally, there is evidence to suggest that the technique fails to label myelinated axons (Somogyi & Smith, 1979; Wouterlood & Mugnani, 1984).

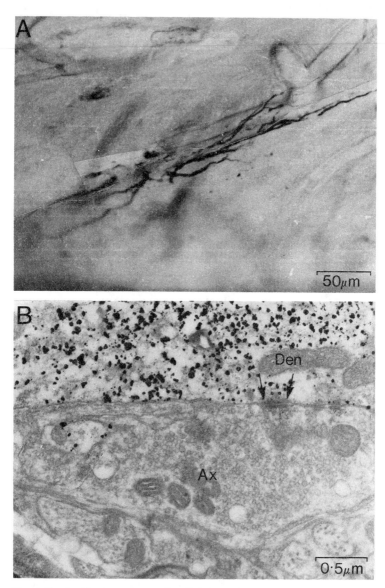

Fig. 1.5 A, Photomontage of a Golgi–gold-toned neurone in lamina I of the spinal cord. B, An electron micrograph illustrating a dendrite (Den) of a gold-toned neurone. Note the particles of metallic gold. Ax = an axon terminal presynaptic to the labelled dendrite (arrows indicate synapse).

1.7 Combined techniques

The majority of methods described can be combined with one or more of the others. This approach offers great scope for the elucidation of neuronal circuits. Combined anatomical techniques become doubly powerful if taken to the ultrastructural level; it is only at this level that synaptic interactions between labelled neurones can firmly be established. As it is not possible to provide an exhaustive review of the many possibilities that combined anatomical studies offer, five examples of studies illustrating the combined approach have been selected from the literature.

Example 1. This is a combination of retrograde tracing with fluorescent dyes and immunocytochemistry (Dalsgaard *et al.*, 1982). In this study the authors wished to demonstrate that primary sensory neurones containing substance P projected to the inferior mesenteric ganglion. They injected True Blue or propidium iodide into the inferior mesenteric ganglion and examined dorsal-root ganglion cells (L2 and L3) for evidence of retrograde labelling. Dorsal-root ganglia were then processed to reveal substance P immunoreactivity and some retrogradely labelled neurones were also found to contain substance P. Therefore they were able to conclude that substance P-containing neurones formed a sensory projection to the inferior mesenteric ganglion.

Example 2. This combination is of retrograde labelling with HRP and intracellular staining (Maxwell *et al.*, 1985). In this series of experiments the authors wished to demonstrate monosynaptic connections between physiologically characterised primary afferent fibres and neurones with axons ascending the dorsal columns of the spinal cord. They retrogradely labelled these neurones by implanting a pellet of HRP into a lesion of the dorsal columns (Enevoldson *et al.*, 1984) and intra-axonally labelled primary afferent fibres using the HRP intracellular staining technique. Neurones receiving contacts from primary afferent fibres could be observed with the light microscope (Figure 1.6A and B) and electron microscopy of contacts revealed that they were synapses. Therefore the authors were able to show conclusively that certain types of primary afferent axons formed monosynaptic connections with this class of neurone.

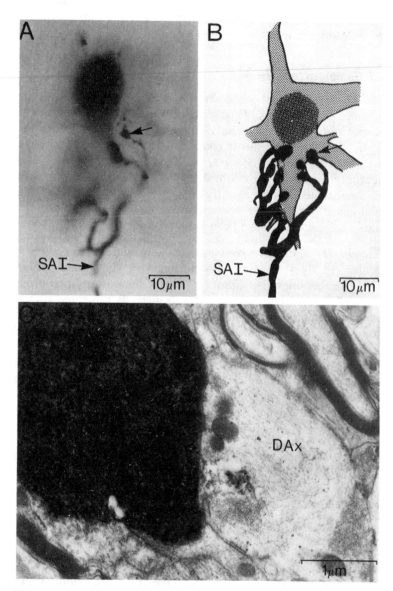

Fig. 1.6 A, Contacts between an intra-axonally HRP-labelled slowly adapting (type 1) primary afferent fibre (SAI) and a postsynaptic dorsal column neurone retrogradely labelled with HRP. Arrow indicates a contact. B, A camera lucida drawing of the structures shown in A. C, An electron micrograph of a dendrite of an intracellularly HRP-labelled spinocervical tract cell and a degenerating primary afferent bouton (DAx).

Example 3. A combination of retrograde HRP labelling, immunocytochemistry and the Golgi technique (Freund *et al.*, 1984) was used in this correlated light and electron microscopical study. The authors wished to examine synaptic contacts formed by tyrosine hydroxylase–immunoreactive boutons with identified striatonigral neurones in the neostriatum. Striatonigral neurones were identified by retrograde labelling with horseradish peroxidase and their dendritic processes were revealed using the section–Golgi procedure (Freund & Somogyi, 1983). The section–Golgi procedure involves reconstitution of a block for Golgi-impregnation from sections processed for HRP and/or immunocytochemistry and can be used in conjunction with light and electron microscopy. Sections to be processed for the Golgi technique were also immunostained to reveal tyrosine hydroxylase. The authors were able to demonstrate synaptic contacts between immunoreactive boutons and spines and dendritic shafts of striatonigral neurones.

Example 4. This is a combination of anterograde degeneration and intracellular staining (Maxwell *et al.*, 1984b). The authors wished to identify boutons originating from primary afferent fibres in contact with physiologically characterised cells (spinocervical tract neurones) in the spinal cord. Dorsal rhizotomies were performed to allow degeneration of primary afferent terminals and spinocervical tract neurones were identified by antidromic stimulation of their axons prior to intracellular labelling with HRP. Under the electron microscope, primary afferent boutons displayed filamentous degeneration and those contacting dendrites of spinocervical tract neurones could readily be identified (Figure 1.6C). Thus the authors were able to identify boutons forming monosynaptic contacts with the projection cells.

Example 5. A combination of intracellular staining and immunocytochemistry (Somogyi & Soltés, 1986) was used by these authors who wanted to demonstrate that basket and clutch cells in the cat's visual cortex contained γ-aminobutyric acid (GABA). Cells were intracellularly labelled and prepared for electron microscopy. Thin sections were immunostained with an antiserum raised against GABA using a post-embedding immunogold procedure. The authors were able to demonstrate concentrations of gold particles over HRP-labelled basket and clutch cell boutons and hence that they contained GABA.

1.8 Concluding remarks

Modern neuroanatomical techniques, whether applied singly or in combination, are greatly increasing our understanding of the central nervous system. They have enabled us to emerge from an era of single-cell analysis to a new era of circuit analysis. They may equally be applied to the normal nervous system, the developing nervous system, the regenerating nervous system or the diseased nervous system; the possibilities are manifold. We have been offered a new set of keys; it is up to us to unlock the secrets that the nervous system holds!

1.9 Further reading

(Other literature is listed in the compiled references at the end of the book.)

Bishop, G. A. & King, J. S. (1982). Intracellular horseradish peroxidase injections for tracing neuronal connections. In: *Tracing Neuronal Connections with Horseradish Peroxidase*, ed. M-M. Mesulam, pp. 185–247. John Wiley & Sons, New York.

Brown, A. G. (1981). *Organization in the Spinal Cord*. Springer-Verlag, Berlin, Heidelberg, New York.

Brown, A. G. & Fyffe, R. E. W. (1984). *Intracellular Staining of Mammalian Neurones*. Academic Press, London.

Cajal, S. Ramon y (1909). *Histologie du système nerveux de l'homme et des vertébrés*. Instituto Cajal, Madrid.

Cowan, W. M., Gottlieb, D. I., Hendrickson, A. E., Price, J. C. & Woolsey, T. A. (1972). The autoradiographic demonstration of axonal connections in the central nervous system. *Brain Research*, **37**, 21–51.

Cuello, A. C. (1983). *Immunohistochemistry*. John Wiley & Sons, New York.

De Mey, J. (1983). A critical review of light and electron microscopic immunocytochemical techniques used in neurobiology. *Journal of Neuroscience Methods*, **7**, 1–18.

Golgi, C. (1873). Sulla struttura della sostanza griga dell cervello.

Gazetta Medica lombarda, **33**, 244–6.

Heimer, L. & Robards, M. J. (1981). *Neuroanatomical tract-tracing methods*. Plenum, New York and London.

Heitler, W. J. (1984). Computer-aided 3-dimensional reconstructions of stained neurones viewed in wholemount. *Journal of Electrophysiological Techniques*, **11**, 87–107.

Kater, S. B. & Nicholson, C. (1973). *Intracellular Staining in Neurobiology*. Springer-Verlag, Berlin, Heidelberg, New York.

Kristensson, K. & Olsson, Y. (1971). Retrograde axonal transport of protein. *Brain Research*, **29**, 363–5.

Kuypers, H. G. J. M., Catsman-Berrevoets, C. E. & Padt, R. E. (1977). Retrograde axonal transport of fluorescent substances in the rat's forebrain. *Neuroscience Letters*, **6**, 127–35.

La Vail, J. H. & La Vail, M. M. (1972). Retrograde axonal transport in the central nervous system. *Science*, **176**, 1416–7.

Mesulam, M.-M. (1982). *Tracing Neuronal Connections with Horseradish Peroxidase*. John Wiley & Sons, New York.

Pitman, R. M. Tweedle, C. D. & Cohen, M. J. (1972). Branching of central neurones: intracellular cobalt injections for light and electron microscopy. *Science*, **176**, 412–4.

Rogers, A. W. (1979). *Techniques in autoradiography*. Elsevier, North Holland.

Sawchenko, P. E. & Gerfen, C. R. (1985). Plant lectins and bacterial toxins as tools for tracing neuronal connections. *Trends in Neurosciences*, **8**, 378–84.

Stewart, W. W. (1978). Functional connections between cells as revealed by dye-coupling with a highly fluorescent napthalamide tracer. *Cell*, **14**, 741–59.

Stretton, A. O. W. & Kravitz, E. A. (1968). Neuronal geometry: determination with a method of intracellular dye injection. *Science*, **162**, 132–4.

Trojanowski, J. Q. (1983). Native and derivatised lectins for *in vivo* studies of neuronal connections and neuronal cell biology. *Journal of Neuroscience Methods*, **9**, 185–204.

van den Pol, A. (1984). Colloidal gold and biotin–avidin conjugates as ultrastructural markers for neural antigens. *Quarterly Journal of Experimental Physiology*, **69**, 1–33.

Zipster, B. & McKay, R. (1981). Monoclonal antibodies distinguish identifiable neurones in the leech. *Nature*, **289**, 549–54.

2

Electrical synapses

W. J. Heitler The Gatty Marine Laboratory, University of St
Andrews

2.1 Introduction

Electrical synapses are sites of neurone-to-neurone communication where the signal is transmitted by the direct flow of current from one cell to the other. This is usually achieved by way of tubular protein bridges (sometimes called 'connexons') which span the extracellular space and provide continuity between the intracellular regions of the pre- and postsynaptic neurones. In the simplest cases an electrical synapse is equivalent to a sudden narrowing in neuronal diameter. Current of either polarity can propagate through such a synapse, with attenuation and delay dependent on the number of connexons present. If there is a potential difference between the two neurones, such as when an action potential (spike) or postsynaptic potential occurs in one of them, mobile ions within the cytoplasm (mainly potassium) tend to flow through the connexons to equilibrate the potentials. The synapse is thus excitatory on the less depolarised neurone, and inhibitory on the more depolarised neurone. However, at more complex electrical synapses the connexons can be gated in either a chemical- or voltage-dependent manner. The flow of ions through such synapses can be regulated, and they are therefore potential sites for circuit modulation.

The connexons are usually large enough to allow small molecules (1–1.5 kD) as well as ions to pass, and thus they provide a means for transmitting metabolites and chemical messengers between the cells. Similar connexons are found in a large range of non-excitable tissues and are presumed to play an important role in chemical communication between cells. In this review I intend to concentrate on the electrical aspects of neuronal communication, but will make occasional forays into non-neural tissue. The essay is aimed at the physiologist who is not already an expert in electrical synapses, does not particularly wish to become an expert in electrical synapses, but would like to be aware of some of the current topics in the field. I refer the reader in search of more specialist knowledge to the book arising from a recent Cold Spring Harbor symposium (edited by Bennett and Spray, 1985), and/or the 'special topic' section of a recent *Annual Review of Physiology* (also edited by Spray, 1985).

2.2 General principles

2.2.1 *How do you know when a synapse is electrical?*

The only absolute criterion for determining the presence of an electrical synapse between two neurones is the demonstration of a low-resistance pathway connecting the interiors of the two cells (Figure 2.1).

This is most satisfactorily achieved experimentally by using microelectrodes to inject a current pulse into one of them, and showing a very short latency voltage perturbation in the second neurone of the same sign as the injected current. The first clear physiological demonstration of an electrical synapse used just this protocol in the crayfish (Furshpan & Potter, 1959). There are four sets of giant fibres (GFs) running the length of the crayfish ventral nerve cord (Figure 2.2), two medial (MG) and two lateral (LG). In the anterior ganglia of the abdomen, these each synapse onto a bilateral pair of powerful abdominal flexor motoneurones called the motor giants (MoGs). The latency of orthodromic transmission across the synapse is about 0.1 ms, (compared to the 0.3–0.5 ms latency typical of chemical synapses). Sub-threshold depolarising (positive) current injected into the presynaptic GF spreads orthodromically to the postsynaptic MoG, while hyperpolarising (negative) current injected into the postsynaptic neurone spreads antidromically into the presynaptic neurone. However, hyperpolarising current does not spread orthodromically, and depolarising current does not spread antidromically. This particular synapse is thus *rectifying* (Figure 2.1C). A similar protocol was used to demonstrate a *non-rectifying* electrical synapse between the LGs themselves (Figure 2.1B). These

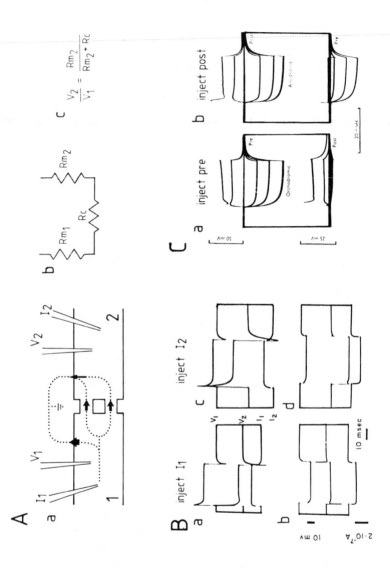

A

a

I_1 V_1 V_2 I_2

1 2

b

Rm_1 Rm_2

Rc

c

$$\frac{V_2}{V_1} = \frac{Rm_2}{Rm_2 + Rc}$$

B

a inject I_1 **c** inject I_2

V_1
V_2
I_1
I_2

b **d**

10 mV 2·10⁻⁷A

10 msec

C

a inject pre **b** inject post

50 mV

Pre Post

Orthodromic

25 mV

Post Pre

Antidromic

Pre

20 msec

bilaterally-paired segmental neurones form a ladder-like network within the abdominal nerve cord but, because of their interconnections by electrical synapses, act like a single neurone (Watanabe & Grundfest, 1961). Things may not always be this simple. Current can *appear* to pass from one cell to the other at a chemical synapse where the presynaptic neurone releases transmitter in a graded manner in response to sub-threshold depolarisation, or even at resting potential (e.g. Burrows, 1980; Graubard *et al.*, 1983; and see Chapter 4). A number of criteria can be used to distinguish this situation from an electrical synapse, but each has potential problems associated with it. Thus a chemical synapse should have a longer delay than an electrical synapse, but unless the electrodes can be placed very close to the synaptic site this may not be detectable. Individual chemical synapses are unidirectional, but reciprocal chemical synapses exist. A chemical synapse with graded transmission should eventually 'bottom out' with sufficient presynaptic hyperpolarisation when all transmitter release is prevented, but the membrane properties of an electrical synapse may produce a similar effect (see below). Finally, the postsynaptic potential of a chemical synapse should have a reversal potential, while the potential generated by an electrical synapse should be impossible to reverse. But this process too is fraught with difficulty, since delayed rectification and/or spike generation, may

---

Fig. 2.1 Basic characteristics of electrical synapses. A(a), A diagram showing a typical experimental procedure for demonstrating electrical coupling, with two microelectrodes inserted on either side of the synapse. A(b), Current injected through one electrode takes one of two paths to ground – across the presynaptic membrane resistance (R_{m1}), or across the synaptic resistance (R_c) and the postsynaptic membrane resistance (R_{m2}). A(c), The coupling coefficient is dependent on R_c and R_{m2} (assuming the electrode V_1 is close to the junction). B, Electrical coupling at the crayfish non-rectifying LG septate synapse: depolarising (a,c) and hyperpolarising (b,d) current pass in either direction across the synapse. C, Electrical coupling at the crayfish rectifying GF–MoG synapse: depolarising but not hyperpolarising current passes orthodromically (a), while hyperpolarising but not depolarising current passes antidromically (b). (B, is modified from Watanabe & Grundfest, 1961; C is modified from Furshpan & Potter, 1959.)

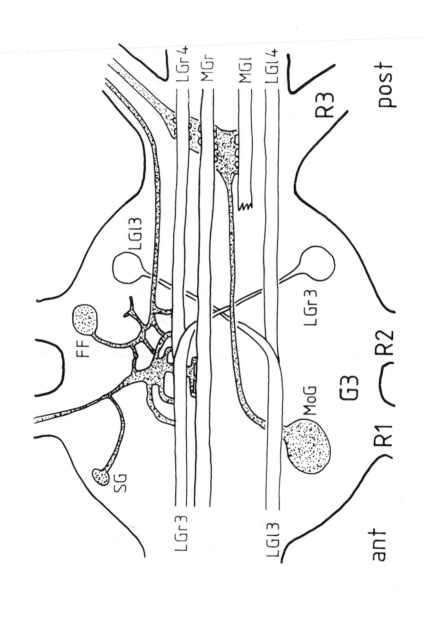

limit postsynaptic depolarisation, while the electrical synapse itself may be voltage-gated.
The problems are exacerbated when dealing with small cells or cells which cannot be easily visualised. In such cases multiple microelectrode placements may not be possible, and indirect evidence must be adduced.

(i) *Dye coupling.* A marker molecule such as Lucifer Yellow of molecular weight 450 (Stewart, 1978; and see Chapter 1) is injected into one cell, and its presence detected in the putative postsynaptic cell. However, false-positive results can occur if neurones other than the intended target cell pick up dye due to damage (the infamous 'shish-kebab' effect). False-negative results are also possible, when neurones which are electrically coupled by physiological criteria fail to show dye-coupling (e.g. Audesirk *et al.*, 1982; Powell & Westerfield, 1984).

(ii) *Response to synaptic uncouplers.* Electrical synapses should be resistant to the usual agents which block chemical synapses (low calcium, high magnesium, cobalt, cadmium, etc.), while they may be susceptible to other agents (intracellular acidification, elevated levels of intracellular calcium, etc., see below).

(iii) *Frequency response.* Many chemical synapses fatigue when stimulated at greater than about 50 Hz, whereas electrical synapses usually do not.

Fig. 2.2 A semi-diagrammatic drawing of the efferent circuitry driving the crayfish escape tail-flip in an anterior abdominal ganglion (G3). Anterior (ant) is to the left, posterior (post) to the right. LG = lateral giant neurone (LGr3 = right-hand LG of G3, etc.); MG = medial giant neurone; MoG = motor giant neurone; SG = segmental giant neurone; FF = fast flexor motoneurone, R1,2,3 = first, second, third roots. Electrical synapses with the specified properties occur between the following sets of neurones;

LG3 – LG4 (the septate synapse): non-rectifying, strong;
LG1 – LGr (the cross-over synapse): non-rectifying, medium;
LG/MG – MoG: rectifying, strong;
LG/MG – SG: rectifying, strong;
SG – FF: probably rectifying, medium;
LG/MG – FF: unknown rectification, weak.

(iv) *Ultrastructure*. Both chemical and electrical synapses have characteristic anatomical features. However, these are not always as clear-cut as the textbooks might lead one to believe (see anatomy section below), and anyway there are often problems in assessing the *functional* significance of ultrastructural features.

It should by now be obvious that in many real experimental situations it can be difficult to be absolutely sure about the nature of a particular synaptic connexion. A nice example of this comes from the locust visual system. Two neurones (the lobular giant movement detector and the descending contralateral movement detector) were originally thought to be connected by an electrical synapse (O'Shea & Rowell, 1975). The evidence was high frequency following (320 Hz), resistance to low calcium and resistance to cooling. However, it was later claimed that the synapse was chemical (Rind, 1984). The evidence for this view was failure to obtain current coupling (there is a presynaptic threshold of 13 mV before a postsynaptic response is obtained and antidromic transmission does not occur), synaptic latency of 1 ms, and a conductance increase in the postsynaptic neurone. The weight of physiological evidence thus leans towards chemical transmission. However, an electron microscope study of the synapse revealed structures characteristic of both chemical *and* electrical synapses (Killmann & Schurmann, 1985).

2.2.2 *How do you quantify electrical synapses?*
The most straightforward form of quantification routinely applied to electrical synapses is the 'coupling coefficient'. This is defined as the ratio of the postsynaptic voltage to the unit presynaptic voltage. In crayfish the non-rectifying electrical synapses connecting the LGs of adjacent ipsilateral segments (the *septate* synapses) have coupling coefficients of 0.3–0.6 (Watanabe & Grundfest, 1961). In this case the coefficients are not significantly different whether measured with relatively long-duration experimentally-applied voltage perturbations, or short-duration voltage pulses resulting from spikes. In contrast, at the rectifying LG–MoG synapse, coupling coefficients are approximately 40% lower for the higher frequency signals (Furshpan & Potter, 1959).

This low-pass filter characteristic is presumably due to the post-synaptic capacitance. Both these sets of synapses normally transmit spikes 1:1.

Coupling coefficients are a useful functional description of the strength of an electrical synapse, but they do not quantify the actual conductance of the connexons mediating the electrical synapse. For a given presynaptic voltage, the postsynaptic voltage will depend on the amount of current passing through the connexons (which is the synapse-specific factor), *and* on the post-synaptic membrane resistance over which this current passes on its way to the extracellular current sink. The actual junctional resistance can be obtained from the measured input resistances of the two neurones and the transfer resistance of the synapse (Bennett, 1966). Alternatively, if the two neurones can be voltage-clamped independently to a common holding potential, then the current required to maintain the clamp in one cell when the other is voltage stepped gives a direct measure of the trans-junctional current. The junctional resistance is thus obtained from Ohms Law (Spray *et al.*, 1981).

2.3 Function of electrical synapses

Electrical synapses are traditionally regarded as having two important functions: speed of transmission and synchronisation of activity. Neuroethological studies certainly support these roles but suggest that the situation is not always so straightforward.

2.3.1 *Speed of response*

Electrical synapses have been found in escape circuitry in animals as diverse as fish (Auerbach & Bennet, 1969), flies (Tanouye & Wyman, 1980) and earthworms (Brink & Barr, 1977), but by far the best worked-out escape system is that of the crayfish tail-flip (reviewed in Wine, 1984). In this circuit nearly every synaptic level is, at least in part, electrical (Figure 2.2). Thus primary tactile afferents on the abdomen of the crayfish make mono-synaptic electrical inputs to the LGs (Zucker, 1972). (They also make chemical inputs to sensory integrating interneurones, which in turn make electrical inputs to the LGs.) The segmental LGs are themselves electrically coupled into a ladder-like chain. The

LGs make electrical output synapses to two neurones in each hemiganglion, the MoG, and the segmental giant neurone (Roberts *et al.*, 1982). The MoG is a specialised motoneurone which causes a large twitch contraction of the fast flexor muscles of the abdomen. The segmental giant is a functional interneurone which excites the non-giant fast flexor motorneurones and a number of swimmeret motoneurones, again through electrical synapses (Roberts *et al.*, 1982; Heitler *et al.*, 1985; Heitler & Darrig, 1986). Thus, other than the chemical output that the primary afferents make to the sensory integrating interneurones, and the chemical output that the motoneurones make at the neuromuscular junctions, every synaptic stage is electrical in this circuit.

2.3.2 *Common activity*

There are numerous examples in the literature of electrical synapses occurring between neurones whose membrane potentials tend to change in parallel. Indeed, this is an inevitable consequence of electrical coupling in its simplest form. In the frog spinal cord, motoneurones innervating the same muscle are electrically coupled, and thus activation is shared between members of the motor pool (Westerfield & Frank, 1982; Collins, 1983). In cardiac pacemaker cells nexi, which are equivalent to electrical synapses, ensure synchronous firing (Torre, 1976). Similarly, a group of endogenous burster neurones in the snail *Lymnaea* are electrically-coupled and fire synchronous spikes. Synchronicity in this case is brought about in part by the electrical excitatory postsynaptic potential (EPSP) resulting from a presynaptic spike resetting the spike-generating mechanism of the post-synaptic cell (Egelhaaf & Benjamin, 1982). In the lobster stomatogastric ganglion a single endogenous burster neurone (AB) is electrically coupled to two non-bursters (the PDs). The coupling is sufficient to ensure that the PDs, too, act like endogenous bursters, and originally they were thought to share this property. It was not until the AB neurone was specifically killed using photoinactivation that it was realised that this was not the case (Miller & Selverston, 1982).

As well as simply tending to synchronise membrane potential changes in coupled neurones, electrical synapses can also bring about emergent network properties. Thus coupling between a group of neurones can in theory cause bursting even when none of the cells is itself an endogenous burster (Getting & Willows, 1974). If one of a group of coupled cells is depolarised and spikes, the electrical EPSPs in the postsynaptic coupled cells will tend to make them spike too. If this happens, they feed back excitation to the first cell, which increases its firing. The postspike hyperpolarisation which would normally follow each spike is reduced because it is shunted away into the coupled cells. The end result is that all the cells tend to fire an accelerating burst of spikes as they mutually excite each other, and the spikes tend to synchronise. The mutual excitation may be augmented by a form of facilitation if the spikes broaden with repetition (see also Chapter 3) and the electrical synapses act as low-pass filters. When the spikes finally do synchronise the mutual excitation ceases. Furthermore, the postspike hyperpolarisation is no longer shunted, since all the neurones in the group are equipotential, having fired synchronously. The burst thus terminates.

Electrical synapses do not always lead to synchronisation, since their effects may depend on their spatial relationship to other synaptic inputs. The oculomotor neurones of teleost fish are electrically coupled through synapses located near the cell bodies. When the neurones are activated through chemical synapses impinging in this region, they fire synchronously, probably mediating rapid behaviours such as saccadic eye movements and eye withdrawal. However, if input synapses activate the neurones at sites of spike initiation remote from the cell body the neurones do not fire synchronously, and smoothly graded nerve volleys can be generated which may be used in slow eye movements (Kriebel *et al.*, 1969).

It is somewhat surprising to find that in some systems neurones are both electrically coupled *and* mutually inhibitory (e.g. the stomatogastric ganglion of lobsters; Mulloney & Selverston, 1974). In this case whether the neurones fire in phase or in anti-phase depends on the relative strengths of the synapses. Since both chemical and electrical synapses can be modulated by extrinsic factors (see below) this sort of circuitry introduces considerable potential plasticity (Marder, 1984).

Finally, in some neural systems the functional importance of

electrical synapses may not be the electrical signal that they pass
but rather some form of chemical signal (Dunlap *et al.*, 1987).
Bioluminescent cells in the hydrozoan coelenterate *Obelia* emit
light in response to an increase in internal calcium concentration.
However, the photocytes themselves do not have calcium channels in their membranes. Instead, the calcium enters *adjacent*
support cells which produce calcium-dependent action potentials.
Light emission is triggered by calcium entering the photocytes
from the support cells by way of electrical synapses.

2.4 Control of electrical synaptic conductance

Although it is probably true that electrical synapses are less
subject to modulation than chemical synapses, it is becoming
increasingly clear that signal transmission through these synapses
is by no means invariant. Two sorts of conductance control may
be distinguished: the first originating from the internal environment of the coupled cells; and the second originating from some
external influence.

2.4.1 Internal control of conductance

The simplest form of conductance control is low-pass frequency
filtering, which nearly all electrical synapses exhibit to some
degree. We have already noted that this can bring about a form
of facilitation. It can also make the PSP resulting from a presynaptic spike biphasic, or even predominantly inhibitory. This
occurs if the rapid depolarising phase of the spike is filtered out,
while the slower after-hyperpolarisation is transmitted (Getting &
Willows, 1974).

Another obvious form of conductance control is rectification.
At the much-discussed crayfish GF–MoG synapse the coupling
coefficient is dependent on transjunctional voltage (Giaume &
Korn, 1983, 1984). In the resting state the GF has a membrane
potential about 15 mV negative to that of the MoG. In this
condition the synapse has a relatively low coupling coefficient of
approximately 0.1. Any increase in this polarisation, as would
occur with an attempt to pass depolarising current antidromically,
decreases the coupling still further. However, if current is injected into either neurone so as to abolish the standing polarisation, the coupling coefficient increases to 0.25, while if the

polarisation is inverted to +37 mV, the coefficient increases to about 0.5. In this condition current of either polarity will pass in either direction across the synapse, and thus the rectification is abolished (Figure 2.3A). Experiments in which both the GF and MoG were cannulated and voltage clamped (Jaslove & Brink, 1986) have shown that the synaptic conductance is controlled by voltage-dependent gates which open and close with a finite time course, as opposed to some sort of instantaneous diode mechanism. At room temperature, the gating is very fast but it slows considerably with cooling. At low temperature, measurements of the current–voltage relationship made *immediately* after a voltage step (i.e. before the channels have time to open or close) are linear in both directions, showing that there is no instantaneous rectification.

The generality of the gate mechanism for rectification is not known, although a similar standing polarisation has been described at rectifying electrical synapses in vertebrates (Auerbach & Bennett 1969). However, within the crayfish itself the electrical synapse from the GFs to the segmental giant neurone is also rectifying but there is no standing polarisation (Heitler & Darrig, 1986). This synapse might simply be at rest in a different part of the polarisation–conductance curve, or a different rectification mechanism might operate. Such different mechanisms certainly exist, since electrical synapses in developing amphibian embryos are also voltage-dependent, but in this case an increase in transjunctional voltage of *either* polarity causes a decrease in coupling coefficient from about 0.8 to 0.1 (Spray *et al.*, 1979). The time course of conductance change is much slower than in the neural tissue, but it too appears to result from the all-or-none gating of individual channels, rather than graded changes in the conductance of a mass of channels (Verselis *et al.*, 1986). Yet another type of voltage sensitivity is found in cells of insect salivary glands, where the trans*membrane* potential, rather than the transjunctional potential is important. Thus equal depolarisation (with respect to the external medium) applied to both of a coupled pair of cells decreases their coupling, while equal hyperpolarisation increases it (Obaid *et al.*, 1983). Given these different characteristics it seems very likely that there is a different molecular basis for the various forms of voltage sensitivity.

The function of neural rectification is usually to ensure unidirec-

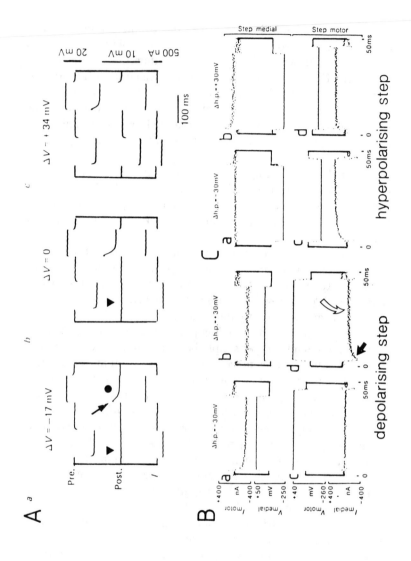

tionality. Thus the motoneurones postsynaptic to the Mauthner cell in the hatchetfish can fire independently of the presynaptic neurone, without any danger of excitation being transmitted back across the synapse (Auerbach & Bennett, 1969). In the crayfish the rectification ensures that the MoG does not act as a coupling neurone between the two sets of GFs. This is functionally very important since the LGs and MGs mediate escape behaviours in opposite directions, so their simultaneous activation would not be a good idea!

Two other features of the internal environment appear to play

---

Fig. 2.3 Mechanism of rectification at the crayfish GF–MoG synapse. A, Orthodromic transmission is dependent on a standing polarisation across the synapse. At rest (a) a depolarising (●) but not hyperpolarising (▲) current pulse is transmitted. (A chemical PSP is also recruited by the depolarisation; arrow.) When the transynaptic polarisation is abolished (b) the depolarising transmission is augmented, but there is still no hyperpolarising transmission. When the polarization is inverted (c) both depolarising and hyperpolarising transmission occurs. The polarisation was altered by constant current injection. B and C, A low-temperature experiment in which both neurones were voltage clamped, first in the low-conductance (negative delta h.p.) state (a,c) and then in the high-conductance (positive delta h.p.) state (b,d). A depolarising (B) and hyperpolarising (C) voltage step (lower trace a,b; upper trace c,d) was applied to the presynaptic MG (a,b) and the postsynaptic MoG (c,d) neurones. The current required to maintain the clamp in the other neurone was measured (upper trace a,b; lower trace c,d).

The records are difficult to interpret for those not used to such data, and so I will describe B in detail. B(a), The junction is initially held at low conductance, but the MG voltage step inverts the polarisation and switches it to high conductance. The current required to clamp the MoG thus starts low but increases as the junctional conductance increases. B(b), The junctional conductance starts high, and the MG voltage step keeps it high, so constant current is required to clamp the MoG. B(c), The junctional conductance starts low, and the MoG voltage step keeps it low. No current is required to clamp MG since none comes through the junction. B(d), The junction is initially high conductance, and thus current is required to maintain the MG clamp after the MoG voltage step (➡). However, this step switches the junction into low conductance, and the amount of current required to maintain the clamp falls (⇨). The time-course of the changing currents is a measure of the time course of the opening and closing of the junctional gates. A is from Giaume & Korn (1984), B and C are from Jaslove & Brink (1986).

a role in determining connexon conductance: the pH and the internal calcium concentration. Elevated internal calcium and internal acidification of the crayfish septate synapse both decrease the coupling coefficient fivefold (Asada & Bennett 1971; Giaume *et al.*, 1980), and similar effects have been observed in a wide range of other tissues (see Spray & Bennett, 1985, for review). The mechanisms of action of pH and calcium are unknown, although in amphibian embryonic cells pH and voltage appear to act on separate gates (Spray *et al.*, 1985). Rapid-freeze fixation of electrically-coupled chick embryo lens epithelial cells has revealed no ultrastructural changes in the connexons specifically associated with changes in conductance (Miller & Goodenough, 1985). Internal perfusion of the crayfish giant axons destroys sensitivity to both calcium and pH (Johnston & Ramon, 1981), and this has been interpreted as indicating that they both act through some soluble intermediary (possibly calmodulin).

The functional significance of this type of uncoupling is not clear. In most cases the changes required to modulate conductance are greater than those occurring under normal conditions (Ramon *et al.*, 1985). An exception might be damaged tissue, where the inflow of calcium from the external medium could induce uncoupling, with obvious consequences for limiting leakage from coupled cells (De Mello, 1983).

2.4.2 *External control of conductance*
External influences may alter the coupling coefficient of an electrical synapse in two ways. Changes in the *non-junctional* membrane resistance of a postsynaptic neurone will produce changes in its voltage response, even if the current coming through the synapse remains constant. Alternatively, changes in the *junctional* resistance itself will produce changes in the synaptic current, and thus alter the postsynaptic voltage response directly. Both these modulating effects have been shown to occur at electrical synapses.

An example of uncoupling by increased extrajunctional conductance comes from the gastropod *Navanax* (Bennet *et al.*, 1985). This animal uses its pharynx in two way: a sudden rapid expansion of the whole organ is used to suck in the prey; while asynchronous contractions are used in peristaltic swallowing and regurgitation. The motoneurones controlling the pharynx are coupled to each other through electrical synapses. This presumably promotes their synchronous firing in the raptorial behaviour. However, tactile stimulation of the pharyngeal wall elicits chemical synaptic input to the motoneurones, resulting in an increase in their input conductance and the total abolition of the electrical coupling. The same sort of stimulus also elicits peristaltic swallowing in which the motoneurones fire asynchronously. Thus the idea is that the electrical coupling can be switched on and off according to the behaviour required. However, it has to be admitted that there is as yet no firm evidence that the animal actually uses this neat mechanism in its real behaviour.

Another example of postsynaptic uncoupling is found in the familiar crayfish GF–MoG rectifying synapse. The MoG can receive a large depolarising chemical IPSP which blocks transmission at the GF–MoG electrical synapse (Wine, 1977). This may be regarded simply as a case of postsynaptic inhibition, but ultrastructural studies have shown that chemical synaptic input seems to be specifically targeted onto dendritic 'bottlenecks' just postsynaptic to the electrical synapse (Stirling, 1972). Synaptic modulation need not always be inhibitory, however, and synaptic inputs which *decrease* the postsynaptic conductance can increase electrical coupling (Carew & Kandel, 1976).

Examples of electrical synapses where external modulators act directly on the junctional conductance are rarer. One case occurs in the horizontal cells of the retina of lower vertebrates (Figure 2.4; Lasater & Dowling, 1985; Neyton *et al.*, 1985). These nonspiking neurones receive hyperpolarising input directly from the photoreceptors and are tightly coupled to each other through electrical synapses. Exogenously applied dopamine reversibly reduces the receptive field of the horizontal cells. Current-coupling and dye-coupling experiments, carried out *in situ* and on isolated cell pairs, both indicate that this change is brought about by a decrease in the junctional conductance *per se* at the electrical synapses. Similar changes were induced by agents which increase intracellular cAMP levels. The conclusion was that dopamine, acting through some cAMP-dependent process, directly effects junctional conductance and hence the size of the horizontal cell receptive field.

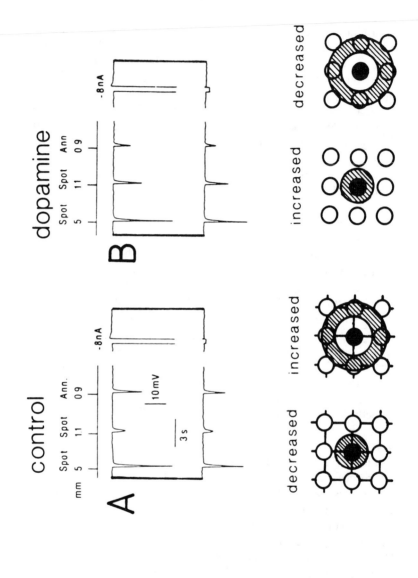

2.5 Anatomy

A structure called the 'gap junction' is widely regarded as the anatomical substrate of an electrical synapse. In thin sections, gap junctions appear as regions where the plasma membranes of adjacent cells are rather smooth and parallel. They come into close apposition but do not fuse; there is an eponymous gap of constant width separating the outer faces. A distinct array of transverse densities spans this gap. In freeze fracture micrographs the densities appear as globules, and a pit or depression 1.2–1.4 nm in diameter is visible in the centre of each. The densities are thought to be tubular and to represent the connexons mediating the coupling.

Examples of gap junctions have been found in virtually every organ in the body of every animal examined. The general features of gap junctions are usually sufficiently distinct for them to

---

Fig. 2.4 Dopamine decreases junctional conductance at electrical synapses between horizontal cells of the turtle retina. Two electrically coupled neurones are recorded simultaneously with microelectrodes. A, Stimuli are presented to a control preparation. The large spot simultaneously stimulates a group of coupled cells, which consequently have an isopotential response so that no current flows through the electrical synapses. The response is thus the 'pure' response of a single cell, unaffected by electrical coupling. The small spot stimulates only a few cells, whose response is attenuated by loss of current through the electrical synapses to adjacent, unstimulated cells. The annulus does not directly stimulate the recorded cells, but these receive current from the surrounding, stimulated cells. Current injected into one cell propagates to the other. The cartoons below the records illustrate these situations for small-spot and annular stimuli (cross-hatching), while recording from a neurone (●) in the centre of a network. A large-spot stimulus (not shown) would cover the whole network in the diagram. B, Identical stimuli are presented after treatment with $5\,\mu\text{mol}\,\text{L}^{-1}$ dopamine. The large spot response is unchanged. The small spot response is increased, since shunting through the electrical synapses is diminished. The annulus response is reduced, since the unstimulated cells no longer receive input from the stimulated cells. The current coupling is marginally increased despite the reduction in junctional conductance. This is presumably because the presynaptic response is strongly increased due to the apparent increase in input resistance. Figure modified from Neyton *et al.* (1985).

be easily recognised but, nonetheless, there is quantitative variation between tissues. The maximum molecular weight which can pass through the junction (presumably a measure of pore diameter) varies between species (Simpson *et al.*, 1977; Flag-Newton *et al.*, 1979). At the crayfish LG septate and GF–MoG synapse the gap separating the opposed membranes is 4–5 nm, the densities are about 10 nm in diameter and the centre-to-centre spacing is about 20 nm (Peracchia, 1973a and b; Hanna *et al.*, 1978; Zampighi *et al.*, 1978). In vertebrates the gap is usually 2–4 nm, the density diameter is 6 nm, and the inter-centre spacing is 8–9 nm (see Table 1 in Zampighi *et al.*, 1978). In both cases the densities are arranged in a polygonal lattice and each density protrudes about 2.5 nm into the cytoplasm of the pre- and post-synaptic axons. A puzzling structural feature found at the crayfish electrical synapses is the presence of vesicles (Figure 2.5). At the LG septate synapse there are clusters of 60 nm vesicles on either side of the apposed membranes. At the GF–MoG and GF-segmental giant synapses there are similar vesicles, but these are located only on the presynaptic side, i.e. in the LG and MG (Zampighi *et al.*, 1978; Hanna *et al.*, 1978; Heitler *et al.*, 1985). Such vesicles are, of course, normally associated with chemical synapses, but there is no physiological evidence that these electrical synapses have any chemical component. The function of the vesicles is at present a mystery but no other structural asymmetry correlating with rectification has yet been found (Hanna *et al.*, 1978).

X-ray diffraction and detailed electron microscope studies suggest that each junction consists of a pair of permeable elements, one from each membrane, tightly jointed in series. The permeable elements contain six subunits arranged as a rosette around a central pore (Makowski *et al.*, 1977; Unwin & Zampighi, 1980; Makowski *et al.*, 1984). Biochemical analysis of the subunits (for review see Revel, 1985) has been hampered by the absence of assays other than electron microscopy, and has been largely carried out on non-neural tissue. There seems to be a single major junctional protein in vertebrate liver gap junctions, and two candidates have been proposed: 'connexin', with a molecular weight of 27 kD (see e.g. Goodenough, 1974; Hertzberg & Gilula, 1979; Finbow *et al.*, 1980), and a 16 kD protein (Finbow *et al.*,

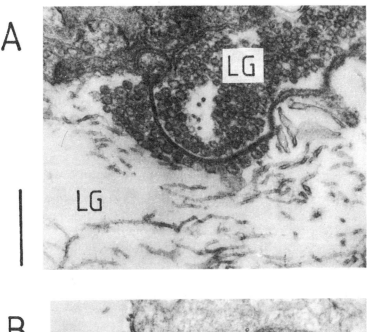

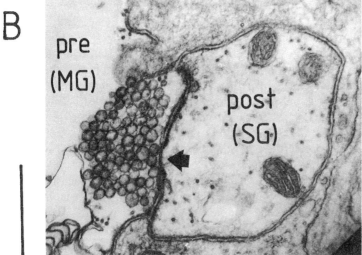

Fig. 2.5 Ultrastructure of electrical synapses in crayfish. A, The non-rectifying septate synapse between the homolateral LGs of adjacent segments: note the close membrane apposition, and the vesicles on either side of the synapse. B, The rectifying synapse between the MG and segmental giant (SG): note the close membrane apposition (arrow), and the vesicles only on the presynaptic side of the synapse. (Scale bars: 500 nm.)

1983). A number of other putative junctional proteins have been isolated from other tissue. Amino acid sequences of junctional protein fragments from heart and liver show reasonable homology, but there is no apparent homology with lens junctional protein (Nicholson *et al.*, 1983). Antibody probes largely confirm these chemical data (for review see Hertzberg, 1985).

2.6 Electrical coupling and development

Gap junctions are particularly widespread in embryos (for review see Caveney, 1985). The coupling is thought to mediate transfer of molecular messengers necessary for embryonic development. Antibodies raised against the 27 kD rat liver gap junction protein have been used to selectively block gap junctions in early amphibian embryos, with disastrous consequences for development (Warner *et al.*, 1984). As development progresses the coupling becomes more restricted. In the locust embryo, neurones derived from different precursors are initially electrically coupled but become uncoupled about half way through embryogenesis (Goodman & Spitzer, 1981). It is interesting that dye uncoupling *precedes* electrical uncoupling, which might imply that the uncoupling process involves the graded closure of individual channels (thus blocking the passage of large dye molecules before that of small ions; *cf.* Verselis *et al.*, 1986). As the axons grow, they become transiently coupled to a variety of 'landmark' cells which seem to guide their development (reviewed in Bastiani & Goodman, 1984). In adult locusts, motoneurones are not normally electrically coupled. An exception to this was a locust where a neurone which normally exists as a single entity was duplicated to form an electrically coupled supernumary pair (Siegler, 1982). This may well have been a case where embryonic coupling persisted into adult life.

Is electrical coupling in the adult nervous system normally a result of the persistence of embryonic coupling? This may be possible when neurones arise from a common precursor and share a common pattern of innervation but it is most unlikely when neurones arise from widely different regions of the nervous system. In *Aplysia* electrical coupling is initially widespread in the embryo but does not persist. The neurones R_2 and $LP1_1$ arise in two different ganglia and are not initially coupled, but they grow axons which form an electrical synapse in a third ganglion (Rayport & Kandel, 1980). Interestingly, this synapse too becomes functionally uncoupled later in the life of the animal; this is a consequence of spatial changes in the relationship between the synapse and the spike initiating site.

Little is known about the processes involved in the developmental formation of electrical synapses, although regenerative changes following damage have been studied. In the snail *Helisoma* neuronal axotomy induces major changes including large amounts of dendritic outgrowth in the region of damage, and changes in neural connectivity. The latter include the formation of entirely new electrical synapses and the strengthening of preexisting electrical synapses (Bulloch & Kater, 1982; Murphey *et al.*, 1983; Cohan *et al.*, 1983). The important point in the *establishment* of a new electrical synapse appears to be that both the neurones involved should be actively growing in the appropriate regions (Hadley & Kater, 1983). Even inappropriate regions of normally uncoupled cells form electrical synapses in culture if they are both growing (Hadley *et al.*, 1982). Some of the novel synapses formed after axotomy are transient and some are permanent. Thus the *stabilisation* of the new synapses appears to be a different process to their initial formation, and as yet no information is available on its control. It is interesting to speculate that the dendritic outgrowth induced by axotomy may represent a return to some sort of pseudoembryological state in which electrical coupling is widespread. The selective elimination of the transient synapses would then be an interesting model for removal of synapses in development.

2.7 Concluding thoughts

We have seen that structures mediating intercellular communication by means of intracellular continuities (gap junctions) are found in a wide range of tissues. In excitable tissues, we assume that in most cases the function of these junctions is *electrical* communication, while in non-excitable tissues *chemical* communication may well be what matters most. Given the differences in protein composition which are being discovered, and the wide range of mechanisms regulating junctional permeability/conductance, it seems likely that not all gap junctions are homologous structures. In the nervous system we are moving away from the idea that electrical synapses only provide invariant, rapid synchronisation of membrane potentials. The properties of frequency filtering, combined with intrinsic and extrinsic control of junctional and near-junctional conductance, suggest that electrical synapses may well display some of the plasticity and modulatability which has previously been thought to be the prerogative of chemical synapses.

2.8 **Further reading**

(Other literature is listed in the compiled references at the end of the book.)

Bastiani, M. J. & Goodman, C. S. (1984). The first growth cones in the central nervous system of the grasshopper embryo. In: *Cellular and Molecular Biology of Neuronal Development*, ed. I. B. Black. Plenum Press, New York.

Bennett, M. V. L. (1966). Physiology of electrotonic junctions. *Annals of the New York Academy of Science*, **137**, 509–39.

Bennett, M. V. L. & Spray, D. C. (1985). *Gap junctions*. Cold Spring Harbor Laboratory, USA.

Bennett, M. V. L., Zimering, M. B., Spira, M. E. & Spray, D. C. (1985). Interaction of electrical and chemical synapses. In: *Gap junctions*, eds. M. V. L. Bennett & D. C. Spray, pp. 355–66. Cold Spring Harbor Laboratory, USA.

Bulloch, A. G. M. & Kater, S. B. (1982). Neurite outgrowth and selection of new electrical connections by adult *Helisoma* neurones. *Journal of Neurophysiology*, **48**, 569–83.

Carew, T. J. & Kandel, E. R. (1976). Two functional effects of decreased conductance EPSP: synaptic augmentation and increased electrotonic coupling. *Science*, 192, 150–3.

Caveney, S. (1985). The role of gap junctions in development. *Annual Review of Physiology*, **47**, 319–35.

Egelhaaf, M. & Benjamin, P. R. (1982). Inhibition by recurrent excitation: a mechanism for spike synchronization in a network of coupled neuronal oscillators. *Journal of Experimental Biology*, **96**, 447–52.

Getting, P. A. & Willows, A. O. D. (1974). Modification of neuron properties by electrotonic synapses. II. Burst formation by electrotonic synapses. *Journal of Neurophysiology*, **37**, 858–68.

Hadley, R. D. & Kater, S. B. (1983). Competence to form electrical connections is restricted to growing neurites in the snail, *Helisoma*. *Journal of Neuroscience*, **3**, 924–32.

Heitler, W. J. & Darrig, S. (1986). The segmental giant neurone of the signal crayfish, *Pacifastacus leniusculus*, and its interactions with abdominal fast flexor and swimmeret motor neurones. *Journal of Experimental Biology*, **121**, 55–75.

Killman, F. & Schurmann, F. W. (1985). Both electrical and chemical transmission between the 'lobula giant movement detector' and the 'descending contralateral movement detector' neurons of locusts are supported by electron microscopy. *Journal of Neurocytology*, **14**, 637–52.

Marder, E. (1984). Roles for electrical coupling in neural circuits as revealed by selective neuronal deletions. *Journal of Experimental Biology*, **112**, 147–67.

Miller, J. P. & Selverston, A. I. (1982). Mechanisms underlying pattern generation in lobster stomatogastric ganglion as determined by selective inactivation of identified neurons. II. Oscillatory properties of pyloric neurons. *Journal of Neurophysiology*, **48**, 1378–91.

Mulloney, B. & Selverston, A. I. (1974). Organization of the stomatogastric ganglion of the spiny lobster. I. Neurons driving the lateral teeth. *Journal of Comparative Physiology*, **91**, 1–32.

Neyton, J., Piccolino, M. & Gerschenfeld, H. M. (1985). Neurotransmitter-induced modulation of gap junction permeability in retinal horizontal cells. In: *Gap junctions*, eds. M. V. L. Bennett & D. C. Spray, pp. 381–91. Cold Spring Harbor Laboratory, USA.

Revel, J-P., Nicholson, B. J. & Yancey, S. B. (1985). Chemistry of Gap Junctions, *Annual Review of Physiology*, **47**, 263–79.

Spray, D. C. (1985). Special topic: gap junctions. *Annual Review of Physiology*, **47**, 261–2.

Spray, D. C., Harris, A. L. & Bennett, M. V. L. (1981). Equilibrium properties of a voltage-dependent junctional conductance. *Journal of General Physiology*, **77**, 75–94.

Stewart, W. W. (1978). Functional connections between cells as revealed by dye-coupling with a highly fluorescent naphthalimide tracer. *Cell*, **14**, 741–59.

Torre, V. (1976). A theory of synchronization of heart pacemaker cells. *Journal of Theoretical Biology*, **61**, 55–71.

Warner, A. E., Guthrie, S. C. & Gilula, N. B. (1984). Antibodies to gap-junctional protein selectively disrupt junctional communication in the early amphibian embryo. *Nature (London)*, **311**, 127–31.

Watanabe, A. & Grundfest, H. (1961). Impulse propagation at the septal and comissural junctions of crayfish lateral giant axons. *Journal of General Physiology*, **45**, 267–308.

Westerfield, M. & Frank, E. (1982). Specificity of electrical coupling among neurons innervating forelimb muscles of the adult bullfrog. *Journal of Neurophysiology*, **48**, 904–13.

Wine, J. J. (1984). The structural basis of an innate behavioural pattern. *Journal of Experimental Biology*, **112**, 283–319.

Zampighi, G., Ramon, F. & Duran, W. (1978). Fine structure of the electrotonic synapse of the lateral giant axons in a crayfish (*Procambarus clarkii*). *Tissue and Cell*, **10**, 413–26.

Zucker, R. S. (1972). Crayfish escape behavior and central synapses. I. neural circuit exciting lateral giant fiber. *Journal of Neurophysiology*, **35**, 599–620.

3

Chemical Synapses

W. Winlow   Department of Physiology, University of Leeds

> The more one finds out about the properties of different synapses, the less grows one's inclination to make general statements about their mode of action.*

3.1 Introduction

Sir Charles Sherrington, one of the founding fathers of the neurosciences, originally coined the term 'synapse' to mean the site at which neurones make functional contact. He did not specify whether this contact was electrical (see Chapter 2) or chemical. Specialised forms of chemical synapses may occur between neurones and muscles (neuromuscular junctions) or between neurones and glands (neuroglandular junctions) and there is great morphological diversity between synapses in the central nervous system. Typically, the presynaptic element of a chemical synapse is filled with synaptic vesicles containing neurotransmitter or neuromodulator substances and is separated from its postsynaptic element by a gap up to 40 nm wide (Figure 3.1A). The postsynaptic membrane is specialised to produce changes in electrical potential when neurotransmitter substances from the presynaptic terminal cross the gap and act on postsynaptic receptor sites. At most chemical synapses synaptic 'noise' occurs, due to spontaneous release of small quantities of transmitter. These are described as miniature endplate potentials (min.epps) at motor endplates (Figure 3.1B), and equivalent events occur at central synapses. When an action potential arrives at a nerve terminal it evokes release of many quanta of transmitter whose effects are

---

* Sir Bernard Katz, *Nerve muscle in Synapse*, 1966.

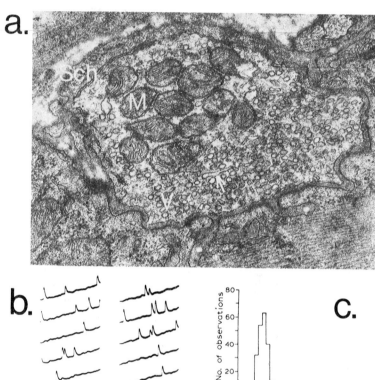

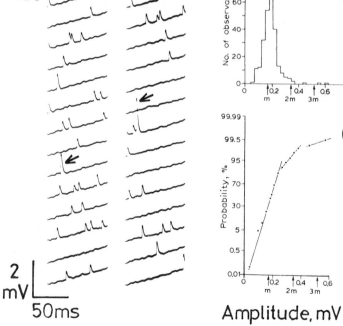

observed in the postsynaptic cell as a smoothly summated post-synaptic potential. In spikeless neurones similar effects may be produced by graded depolarisation of the nerve terminals (see Chapter 4).

3.2 The vesicle hypothesis for transmitter release

The cholinergic vertebrate neuromuscular junction shown in Figure 3.1a has been used for many experiments on synaptic physiology because of its accessibility. Experiments on neuro-muscular junctions, correlated with ultrastructural observations of synaptic vesicles, led many authors to believe that the min. epps were the physiological manifestation of exocytosis of the synaptic vesicles from the presynaptic terminal. This in essence is the vesicle hypothesis, which is shown schematically in Figure 3.2.

Unfortunately, although the vesicle hypothesis is both elegant and appealing it has not been finally established. Many lines of evidence can be shown to support it (Table 3.1) but a number of inconsistencies have been demonstrated (Table 3.2) suggesting that the simple form of the hypothesis may require considerable modification. This raises several questions regarding the release of neurotransmitter substances:

Fig. 3.1 Characteristics of a chemical synapse (motor endplate of mouse diaphragm). (a) Electron micrograph of a motor endplate showing the Schwann cell cap (Sch), large numbers of mitochondria (M) and synaptic vesicles (V) and a terminal cisterna (arrow) from which vesicles are thought to be budded off. (Scale bar = 1 μm.) (b) Miniature endplate potentials (min. epps) recorded from the muscle directly underlying the motor endplate. Min. epps of varying sizes were recorded and a frequency histogram of min. epp amplitudes from another terminal is shown in (c). This has a skewed appearance due to the presence of 'giant' min. epps (attributed to multiquantal release) in the discharge (see arrows in b). (d) Probability plot of the data from (c) gives a series of straight lines suggesting that there are three overlapping normal distributions clustered around multiples of the mean of the first population (m, 2 m and 3 m). At this particular end-plate, 14% of the min. epps were giant min. epps. (Taken from Winlow & Usherwood, 1975, Figure 3.1a and Winlow & Usherwood, 1976, Figure 3.1C and D.)

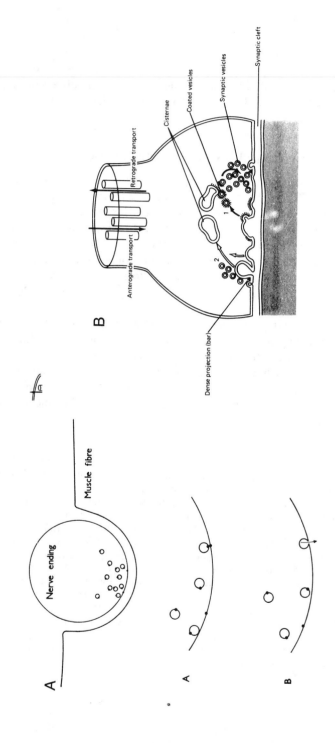

Do vesicles exist, or are they preparation artifacts? According to Gray (1977), vesicles may be artifacts which appear or disappear depending on the preparative procedures for electron microscopy. He further suggests that they may be spheres derived from the break-up of neurotubules. This seems an improbable postulation, since vesicles appear to contain high concentrations of neurotransmitters, which are unlikely to be captured by dissociating neurotubules. A more likely hypothesis is that microtubules are involved in translocation of vesicles to active zones in the presynaptic membrane (Gray, 1978).

If vesicles exist what is their function? Most physiologists would answer this by referring to the vesicle hypothesis and pointing out that the vesicles are very obviously the primary secretory organelle of the presynaptic terminal, but this has proved extremely difficult to demonstrate conclusively. Recent, elegant studies on cultured molluscan neurone cell bodies indicate that

---

Fig. 3.2 The vesicle hypothesis for transmitter release. A, schematic diagram to explain quantal release of transmitter, as a result of critical collision between vesicle and axon membrane, leading to temporary membrane fusion and exocytosis of vesicle contents into the synaptic cleft. Black dots indicate active sites on the surface of the vesicles and on the axon membrane. Transmitter release occurs when active sites on vesicles come into contact with active sites on the axon membrane. In the resting state, successful membrane fusions are comparatively rare and account for synaptic 'noise'. Depolarisation of the terminal by an invading action potential increases the number of active sites and hence the amount of transmitter released. (From Del Castillo & Katz, 1957.) B, two mechanisms for recycling of vesicle membranes are illustrated. In pathway 1 (➡), which is physiologically the most important, excess membrane is selectively retrieved by means of endocytosis of coated pits from the non-active zones of the membrane. The coating on the pits is a specific protein known as clathrin. After a period of activity the area of the presynaptic membrane enlarges and many more coated pits are observable. After endocytosis they pass to membrane cisternae and fuse with them. The cisternae then bud off further synaptic vesicles which are believed to pass back to the preterminal membrane for re-use. The second pathway (⇨) involves endocytosis of uncoated pits from active zones of the membrane. They are formed in the first few seconds after exocytosis, but their function is unclear. (From Kandel & Schwartz, 1985.)

functional chemical synapses may be formed between pairs of spherical cell bodies after a few days (Haydon, 1989). Ultra-structural studies on simple preparations of this sort may help us correlate the first appearance of min epps with the presence or absence of synaptic vesicles. Whatever the outcome, March-banks' hypothesis (1979) that vesicles represent a storage organelle would seem attractive. Perhaps some vesicles store neurotransmitters, whilst others are capable of releasing their contents by exocytosis.

How is transmitter released if not by exocytosis? If transmitter is not released by the process of exocytosis of vesicle contents, another mechanism must be postulated. The alternative mechanism favoured by a number of authors is that of translocation of cytoplasmically stored neurotransmitter through large conductance channels in the presynaptic membrane. This is known as the *cytoplasm-gate hypothesis*. The introduction of the patch–clamp technique, whereby the existence of specific membrane channels can be investigated, recently allowed this hypothesis to be tested at developing neuromuscular junctions between pairs of cultured amphibian nerve and muscle cells (Young & Chow, 1988). Since there was no intervening axon it was thus possible to record simultaneously from both the pre- and postsynaptic cell, but *no evidence for large transmitter channels was demonstrable*, indicating that the cytoplasm-gate hypothesis is probably unsupportable.

A rather more promising hypothesis is the *operator hypothesis*, in which the operator is the functional unit responsible for transmitter release and triggered by calcium entry into the cytoplasm (see section 3.4). Israel *et al.* (1979), suggested three forms of possible operator as shown in Figure 3.3. The saturable gate (Figure 3.3A) is really another form of the cytoplasmic-gate hypothesis and can be discounted immediately, but the idea of *operator vesicles* (Figure 3.3B) or *carrier proteins* (Figure 3.3C) binding fixed amounts of transmitter are attractive and cannot be easily dismissed. Operator vesicles are envisaged as drawing neurotransmitter from cytoplasmic pools and expelling it into the synaptic cleft. The majority of vesicles do not contain newly synthesised transmitter and take up to a day to refill. Thus, if operator vesicles are ever found to exist, they will need to become rapidly saturated with acetylcholine in order to fulfil the role postulated for them.

The role of putative carrier proteins is rather more contentious since it is difficult to see how they could ensure synchronous transfer of fixed amounts of transmitter across the membrane and most such molecules have relatively low turnover rates.

What is the present status of the vesicle hypothesis? According to Jones (1981): 'The vesicle hypothesis in its simple form appears untenable, as the vesicles of the presynaptic terminal are probably not the homogeneous entities once believed.' Perhaps the best compromise is to assume that, at most adult synapses, some vesicles are for storage of transmitter, whilst others (operator vesicles) participate in transmitter release and membrane recycling. Assuming that, in most synapses, exocytosis is the norm for transmitter release, we are left to wonder how transmitter is actually transferred into vesicles in the first instance and how, following recycling, the vesicle and presynaptic membranes resegregate after fusion, since they are structurally distinct from one another.

3.3 Specialisations of the pre- and postsynaptic membranes

The structure of the active zones of the pre- and postsynaptic membranes have been demonstrated by use of the freeze fracture technique and electron microscopy and are summarised in Figure 3.4. The presynaptic terminal contains dense bars on either side of which rows of synaptic vesicles are found to occur, just above a series of intramembranous particles which are thought to be permanent specialisations involved in vesicle discharge. No evidence yet exists but they could represent terminal calcium channels, which have been demonstrated electrophysiologically (see next section). At neuromuscular junctions, postsynaptic receptors are localised on the postjunctional folds and may be represented by the particles shown on the postsynaptic membrane in Figure 3.4.

Table 3.1   *Evidence in favour of the vesicle hypothesis*

Evidence	Source(s)
Presynaptic terminals contain synaptic vesicles	Sjostrand, 1953; Palay, 1954, Palade, 1954
Synaptic vesicles contain neurotransmitters	Many authors: for reviews, see Klein *et al.* 1982
Miniature end-plate potentials (min. epps) are recorded as synaptic 'noise' in the postsynaptic cell	Fatt & Katz, 1952
Min. epp amplitudes fit a Poisson distribution suggesting that they are 'quantal' in nature	Boyd & Martin, 1956
Evoked release of min. epps occurs in multiples of the quantal unit	For review see Martin, 1977
High magnesium saline diminishes evoked transmitter release and leaves synaptic vesicles fused to the presynaptic membrane.	Heuser *et al*, 1971
Degeneration of terminals leads to: (a) loss of synaptic noise as terminals are engulfed by Schwann cells, which subsequently occupy their positions over the postjunctional folds at the neuromuscular junction in some species;	Miledi & Slater, 1968, 1970; Winlow & Usherwood, 1975, 1976
(b) establishment of low frequency min. epp discharges within a few days of denervation, possibly correlated with release of vesicles from engulfed terminals now within the Schwann cells;	Birks *et al.* 1960
(c) bursts of min. epps are correlated with aggregates of vesicles at locust neuromuscular junctions	Rees & Usherwood, 1972a,b
Application of toxins, e.g. black widow spider venom, causes complete loss of vesicles and minepps from neuromuscular junctions, following a short period of greatly enhanced min. epp discharge	Okamoto *et al.*, 1971; Clark *et al.*, 1972

Prolonged stimulation of presynaptic elements leads to depletion of vesicles and increases the area of the presynaptic membrane suggesting addition of material to that membrane	Ceccarelli *et al.*, 1972; Pysh & Wylie, 1972
Recycling of vesicle membranes has been demostrated by use of the extracellular tracer, horseradish peroxidase, which is at first taken up into vesicles via terminal cisternae and then externalised after stimulation	Heuser & Reese. 1973; 1981
Quick-freeze and freeze fracture studies demonstrate exocytosis at the presynaptic membrane, particularly in the presence of 4-aminopyridine, which prolongs action potentials in the presynaptic terminals by selectively blocking potassium channels	Heuser *et al.*, 1979; Fesce *et al.*, 1980
Fusion of synaptic vesicles to presynaptic terminal membranes may be controlled by calcium dependent synaptic vesicle associated proteins	Trimble & Scheller, 1988

Table 3.2   *Evidence against the vesicle hypothesis*

Evidence	Source(s)
At motor endplates and some central synapses only about 50% of acetylcholine is contained in vesicles. The remainder lies in the cytoplasm	Many authors: reviewed by Israel *et al.*, 1979
Min.epps are of variable size	See Israel *et al.*, 1979
Vesicles may be artifacts of fixation of tissue for electron microscopy	Gray, 1975, 1977
The biochemical structure of vesicle membranes differs from that of the cell membrane	Whittaker, 1966; Iversen & Bloom, 1970
Acetylcholine may be directly released into the synaptic cleft from the cytoplasm	Tauc, 1977; Marchbanks, 1977

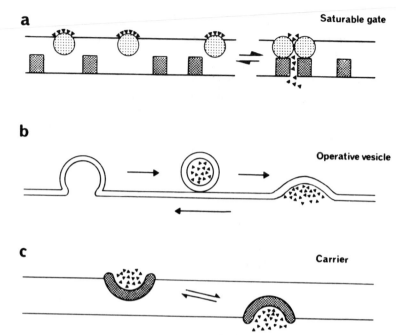

Fig. 3.3 The operator hypothesis for acetylcholine release. Three possible operators for releasing neurotransmitter substances are suggested. (a) The saturable gate: transmitter is bound to membrane proteins which meet complementary proteins to form a transmembrane channel. Recent patch-clamp evidence makes this hypothesis untenable (see text). (b) The presynaptic membrane is recycled, perhaps in the in the way shown in Figure 3.2. The operative vesicles could be a different population from the majority of synaptic vesicles which may act as reserve store. (c) Release is accomplished by carrier proteins able to bind a fixed amount of neurotransmitter. (From Israel *et al.*, 1979.)

3.4 The role of calcium in transmitter release

Whatever the mechanism by which neurotransmitters are released from the presynaptic terminal, calcium is vital for this process to take place (for review see Junge, 1981). Ever since the end of the last century, it has been known that calcium ions are necessary for neuromuscular transmission to take place, but it was not until the 1960s and 1970s that this was shown to be due

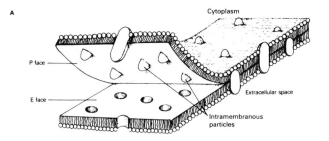

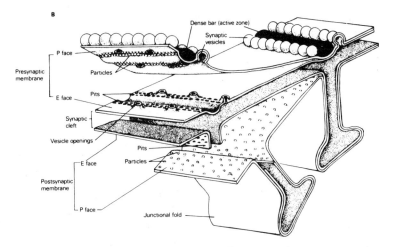

Fig. 3.4 The structure of synaptic membranes at the neuromuscular junction revealed by the freeze fracture technique. A, demonstrates the freeze fracture technique in which the lipid bilayer is split along the hydrophobic interior resulting in two complementary fracture faces: the inner half-membrane or P face contains most of the globular intra-membranous proteins; the outer half membrane or E face contains pits complementary to the protein particles. B, Three-dimensional view of the pre- and postsynaptic membranes showing active zones and synaptic vesicles overlying presynaptic membrane particles. The particles on the P face of the postsynaptic membrane may be postsynaptic receptor sites. (From Kandel & Schwartz, 1985.)

to an effect on the presynaptic membrane. Early studies carried out at the vertebrate neuromuscular junction supported this view. In preparations where the presynaptic action potential was blocked with the specific sodium channel blocker tetrodotoxin (TTX), focal application of calcium to the terminals permitted transmitter release, but only when applied shortly before a depolarising stimulus (Figure 3.5). This implied that external calcium ions entered the axon terminals to trigger transmitter release and that the role of sodium ions was to depolarise the terminal. Further studies on the squid giant synapse confirmed that this was the case. The beauty of this preparation is that both the presynaptic and postsynaptic elements of the synapse are very large and can be penetrated simultaneously with glass microelectrodes for stimulation and recording. Thus the membrane potentials of both neurones may be easily adjusted by current injection through the electrodes.

In the squid giant synapse, action potentials were blocked with TTX, but brief depolarising pulses to the presynaptic terminal produced excitatory postsynaptic potentials (epsps) in the postsynaptic neurone. By also blocking potassium channels with the specific blocking agent tetraethylammonium (TEA), it proved possible to depolarise the terminal to +130mV (the reversal potential for calcium) and totally to suppress the epsps, implicating calcium in transmitter release since no other ion is available under these circumstances. Direct evidence to support the calcium hypothesis for chemical synaptic transmission is derived from experiments in which aequorin, a calcium-sensitive light-emitting protein from jellyfish, was injected into neurones and produced a light signal following repetitive stimulation (Figure 3.6).

3.5 The postsynaptic potential

In the mammalian brain, the vast majority of synapses are thought to be chemical in nature and the transmitter released from an axon terminal by an invading action potential produces a postsynaptic potential (psp) in the postsynaptic cell. Each individual neurotransmitter produces its action on the postsynaptic membrane by acting on specific postsynaptic receptor sites, which are capable of opening gates in specific membrane channels. Particular ionic species pass through particular channels and are driven either into or out of the cell according to their electrochemical gradient. In some cases the physiological stimulus acts directly on the channel protein and directly affects its gating function (Figure 3.7A), whilst in others the sensor (receptor molecule) is physically remote from the channel protein and a diffusible second-messenger protein (e.g. cyclic AMP) is required to open the gate (Figure 3.7B).

Psps may either excite (epsps, which depolarise) or inhibit (ipsps, which hyperpolarise) the postsynaptic cell and in some cases more complex mixed psps occur (see next section). Whatever the case, psps result from ionic currents entering or leaving neurones when ions pass down their electrochemical gradients to produce resultant shifts in membrane potential. Thus, epsps are produced by a net inward movement of positive charge, whilst ipsps are produced by a net outward movement of positive charge, and all psps are produced as a consequence of a conductance change in the postsynaptic membrane.

Originally, all psps were thought to be driven by transient increases in conductance to various ionic species at *conductance increase synapses*. More recently, a number of synapses have been shown to operate using a decreased conductance mechanism and are described as *conductance decrease synapses*. Ionic flows depend on two factors, the electrochemical gradient (i.e. ion concentrations on either side of the cell membrane and the cell-membrane potential) and the membrane conductance for that particular ion. For any particular ion there is an equilibrium potential at which no net flow of ion occurs. If the cell membrane is artificially set to one side of this equilibrium potential current will flow into the cell, but if it is set to the other side of the equilibrium potential, current will flow out of the cell. In Figure 3.8 the two types of synapse are compared with respect to sodium ions, which in the case of a conductance increase synapse produce epsps, but in conductance decrease synapses they produce ipsps. A complete treatment of the ionic mechanisms underlying synaptic transmission is beyond the scope of this chapter and should be sought in Junge (1981), Hille (1984) or Shepherd (1987).

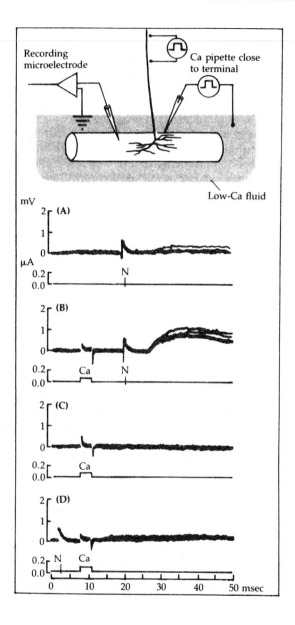

3.6 Neurones with multiple postsynaptic actions

Sherrington first introduced the concept that neurones could have more than one postsynaptic action as long ago as 1906. Unfortunately, he chose to suggest the principle of reciprocal innervation, utilising a single transmitter, for the antagonistic muscles involved in the flexor and extensor reflexes of decerebrate cats and was later proved wrong by Eccles and his coworkers. They demonstrated the presence of an additional interneurone in the inhibitory pathway (see Kandel, 1976, for review). This led Eccles to speculate that a single neurone could only have a single function. Taken together with the suggestion that neurones release only a single transmitter substance from all their terminals (often misleadingly called Dale's principle) the classical view of connections between neurones (Figure 3.9) was that: 'any one class of nerve cells will function exclusively either in an excitatory or an inhibitory capacity at all of its synaptic endings, i.e. there are functionally just two types of nerve cells, excitatory and inhibitory' (Eccles, 1957). The first evidence to the contrary was demonstrated on neurones of the marine mollusc *Aplysia californica* by Strumwasser (1962).

Much of the recent work demonstrating that single neurones can have a multiplicity of postsynaptic actions has been carried out on gastropod molluscs (Kandel, 1976) which have large identifiable neurones. Using this type of preparation, it is feasible

---

Fig. 3.5 The importance of extracellular calcium for transmitter release at the motor endplate. The upper panel shows the arrangements for extracellular stimulation of the main nerve trunk, intracellular recording from the region of the motor endplate and iontophoretic application of calcium from the calcium pipette placed close to the nerve terminals. A, In low calcium solution repeated motor nerve impulses (N) cause little or no transmitter release. B, The nerve impulse is immediately preceded by application of calcium (Ca) to the terminal from the pipette and transmitter is released to produce an endplate potential (epp). Either application of calcium alone (C), or application of calcium after the arrival of nerve impulse, but before the expected epp (D) has no effect on transmitter release. (From Kuffler *et al.* 1984.) This implies that calcium enters the nerve terminal immediately after the arrival of the nerve impulse, probably due to the opening of voltage-dependent calcium channels.

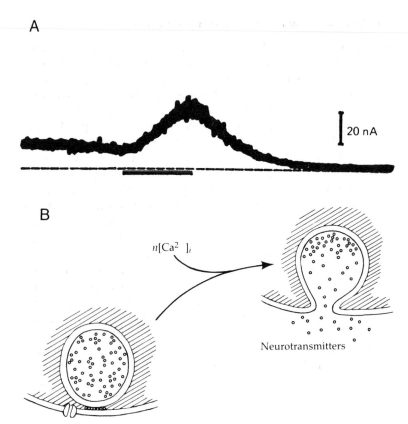

Fig. 3.6   The role of calcium in transmitter release A, Calcium entry
into the presynaptic terminals of a squid giant synapse is demonstrated
following aequorin injection into the presynaptic neurone: upper trace,
light emitted by aequorin during and after a 45 s stimulus pulse (bar).
(From Llinás *et al.* 1972.) B, Illustrates the way in which calcium entry
may trigger release of neurotransmitter substances. Depolarisation at
nerve terminals acts as a secretory signal, which opens voltage-dependent calcium channels. Neurotransmitter is then released after *n*
calcium ions have triggered the necessary membrane fusion and resultant
exocytosis. (From Hille, 1984.)

(A) CHANNEL USING INTRINSIC SENSOR

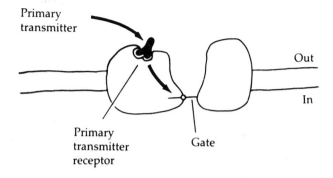

(B) CHANNEL USING REMOTE SENSOR

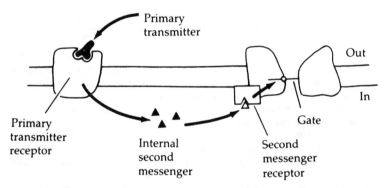

Fig. 3.7 Intrinsic and remote membrane receptors for neurotransmitters. At some membranes the sensor (receptor) for a neurotransmitter acts directly on the channel macromolecule to affect its gating function (as shown in A), whilst in other cases the channel sensor is a physically separate macromolecule (as shown in B). In this case it communicates with the channel macromolecule through a diffusible, intracellular second messenger molecule. (From Hille, 1984.)

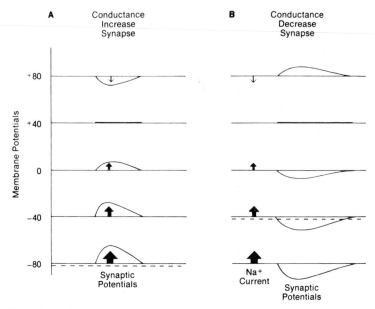

Fig. 3.8 Comparison of conductance-increase and conductance-decrease synapses for sodium ions. Synaptic potential amplitudes are shown at different levels of membrane potential and the arrows indicate the direction and intensity of sodium current flow. At conductance decrease synapses (B), the resting sodium conductance is greater than in conductance increase synapses (A) and the resting membrane potential is therefore lower (---), due to the depolarisation caused by the inward sodium leak. When neurotransmitter is released onto this membrane it decreases sodium conductance, unlike the case in (A) where sodium conductance is increased. Thus in both cases the membrane potential moves towards the equilibrium potential of the ions to which the membrane is most permeable, i.e. depolarisation towards the sodium equilibrium potential in (A) and hyperpolarisation towards the potassium and chloride equilibrium potentials in (B). In both cases the potentials reverse around the sodium equilibrium potential. Note that the time-course of synaptic potentials in (B) is considerably longer than in (A), since decreased conductance raises membrane resistance and increases the membrane time constant, thus slowing down the potential change. Similar mechanisms also exist for potassium ions and slow epsps can be produced by diminishing potassium conductance. (From Shepherd, 1983.)

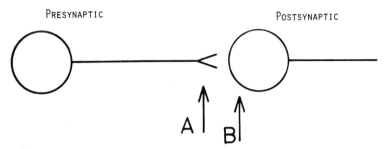

Fig. 3.9 The classical view of neural connections is that a single neurone secretes a single transmitter substance and is capable of only a single postsynaptic action. A, one transmitter (Dale, 1935). B, One postsynaptic action (Eccles, 1957).

to use various criteria for the demonstration of novel monosynaptic connections, many of which cannot be used in the more complex and less easily accessible nervous systems of vertebrates (Figure 3.10). These criteria are summarised in Table 3.3.

Here, the known synaptic connections of a multiaction neurone of the freshwater snail *Lymnaea stagnalis* are used to demonstrate the principle that a single neurone may have several postsynaptic actions. The large dopamine-containing neurone, termed R.Pe.D.1 (right pedal ganglion dorsal neurone 1), inhibits some of its follower cells, excites others, and his biphasic effects on others (Figure 3.11). It fulfills the criteria for monosynaptic transmission set out in Table 3.3. Since the postsynaptic actions of the neurone may be mimicked by iontophoretic application of dopamine to its follower cells, we are driven to the conclusion that the postsynaptic actions of a particular transmitter on a follower cell are determined by the postsynaptic receptors on the follower-cell membrane. Kandel and his co-workers have clearly demonstrated which ion channels can be operated by acetylcholine in follower cells of the interneurone L10 in *Aplysia* (Figure 3.12). Table 3.4 lists examples of neurones with multiple postsynaptic actions.

Clearly Eccles' view that each neurone has a single class of postsynaptic actions is difficult to substantiate on the basis of the evidence presented here, but it is very difficult to disprove in mammalian tissue due to major technical difficulties. However, dual-action neurones have been observed in the parasympathetic

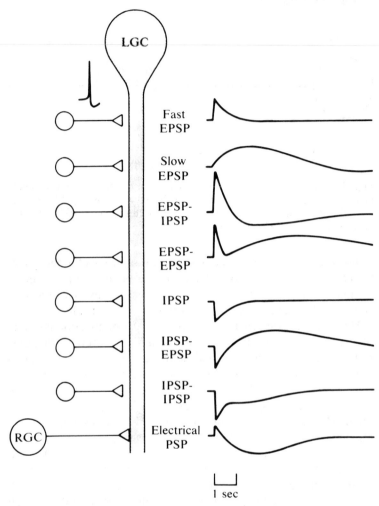

Fig. 3.10 Many different types of unitary postsynaptic potentials exist. Here they are demonstrated on the giant cell of the left pleural ganglion (LGC) of *Aplysia*, by stimulation of a series of different presynaptic interneurones found in the pleural ganglion. Both pure inhibitory and pure excitatory psps are visible as well as various forms of biphasic psps, some of which combine excitatory and inhibitory actions, whilst others combine slow and fast psps of the same polarity. These actions are mediated by a whole variety of neurotransmitters, including dopamine, serotonin and acetylcholine. Thus many different postsynaptic receptors coexist on the same postsynaptic membrane. (From Shimihara & Tauc, 1975.)

Table 3.3 *Popular criteria for monosynaptic connections between identified neurones*

A	1:1 Relationship between presynaptic spike and postsynaptic potential (psp)
B	Constant latency between spike and psp
C	Latency not altered by soaking preparation in high Mg^{2+} saline (reduces transmitter release)
D	Transmission not blocked and latency not altered by soaking preparation in high calcium saline (raises threshold/enhances transmitter release)
E	Amplitude and/or duration of psp is increased by injecting presynaptic cell with tetraethyl ammonium (TEA)

ganglion of the mudpuppy, a primitive amphibian, and goldfish Mauthner cells also have dual actions. Thus individual neurotransmitter substances are capable of a variety of postsynaptic actions. To make the situation yet more complicated, many neurones are now known to contain more than one transmitter substance (e.g. Osborne, 1983). Although the presence of a multiplicity of transmitters, or transmitter precursors, in a neurone does not prove that they are physiologically active compounds, or even that they are secreted from the nerve terminals, the concept that a neurone necessarily contains only one transmitter cannot now be accepted and is discussed in Chapter 7.

3.7 Synaptic plasticity

Many forms of plasticity exist in the nervous system (e.g. Winlow & McCrohan, 1987), but here we are most concerned with mechanisms underlying changes in mobilisation of transmitter release. At many synapses, repetitive stimulation results in a gradual decline of the psp and this phenomenon is described as *synaptic depression*. At other synapses the opposite occurs in that repetitive stimulation of the presynaptic neurone leads to an increase in the amplitude of the psp, known as *synaptic facilitation*. Thus synapses may exhibit *use-dependence* and this may be partly controlled by *prejunctional autoreceptors*, which modify the availability of transmitter in relation to demand via a series

Types of p.s.p. mediated by R.Pe.D.1

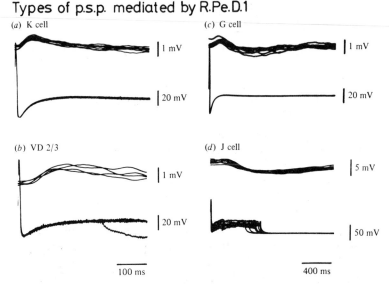

Fig. 3.11 Examples of the different types of psp induced by the giant dopamine containing neurone, R.Pe.D.1 of *Lymnaea*, on its follower cells. In (a) and (c), respectively, examples of epsps with short and long latencies to onset are shown. In (b) and (d), respectively, biphasic and pure inhibitory psps are demonstrated. In each case the sweep of the oscilloscope was triggered from the rising phase of the R.Pe.D.1 action potential. Each panel is made up of a number of superimposed sweeps. Note the difference in time scale for (a) and (c) as compared with (b) and (d). (From Winlow *et al.*, 1981.)

of complex metabolic pathways in the presynaptic neurone (Bowman *et al.*, 1988). These actions were first observed at neuromuscular junctions in crustacea, but similar events occur at central synapses where they may contribute to the learning process. Learning is a complex behavioural event but recent experiments on *Aplysia* reveal that it may be partly due to changes in transmitter mobilisation induced by changes in inward calcium currents.

At a behavioural level, all animals become habituated to the repeated presentation of a non-noxious stimulus. *Habituation* is usually observed as a change in the strength of a reflex response; much of the early work on habituation was carried out on the

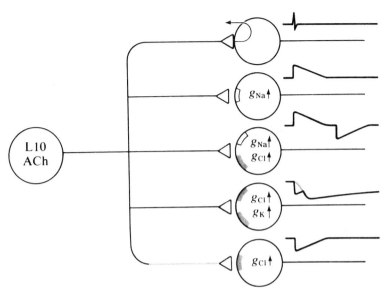

Fig. 3.12 Mediation of different synaptic actions by different branches of the cholinergic interneurone, L10 of *Aplysia*. These actions on different follower cells are shown schematically and include (from top to bottom) biphasic electrical coupling, chemical excitation (mediated by sodium ions), two-component chemical excitation–inhibition (sodium and chloride ions), two-component chemical inhibition (chloride and potassium ions) and chemical inhibition (chloride ions). Thus the same transmitter can have a multiplicity of effects depending on the type of receptors on the postsynaptic neurone. (From Kandel, 1976.)

spinal reflexes of mammals. In *Aplysia*, it has been possible to study the cellular mechanisms underlying habituation in detail, using a simple reflex arc, whereby gentle stimulation of the sensory neurones of the siphon cause a protective withdrawal response of the gill (Figure 3.13A and B) through a monosynaptic pathway to the gill motoneurones (Figure 3.13C). After repeated stimulation the behavioural response declines markedly and current evidence suggests that this habituation is due to a diminution in the number of quanta of transmitter released from the sensory cells, which in turn diminishes the size of the psps in the motoneurones (Kandel & Schwartz, 1982). The primary cellular

Table 3.4 *Summary of some known multiaction neurones*

Animal	Cell	Transmitter	Postsynaptic effect							Reference
			E	EI	EE	I	IE	II	ELEC	
Aplysia	L10	Ach	✓	✓		✓		✓	✓	Kandel et al., 1967 et seq.
Aplysia	BR4	Ach	✓	✓		✓		✓		Gardner & Kandel, 1972 et seq.
Navanax	?	Ach		✓						Levitan & Tauc, 1972
Aplysia/Helix	Metacerebral cells	5-HT	✓		✓	✓				Cottrell, 1970; Cottrell & Macon, 1974; Greschenfeld & Paupardin–Tritsch, 1974
Planorbis	GDC	Dopamine	✓	✓		✓			✓	Berry & Cottrell, 1975, 1979
Lymnaea	R.Pe.D.1 (= RPGN)	Dopamine	✓	✓		✓			?	Winlow & Benjamin, 1977; Winlow et al., 1981
Goldfish	Mauthner cells		✓			✓				Yasargil & Diamond, 1968
Mudpuppy	Principal cells	Ach	✓			✓				Roper, 1976

event governing these changes in transmitter release is a diminution of the number of presynaptic calcium channels opening on arrival of the action potential at the presynaptic terminal.

During the process of *sensitisation*, a reflex is enhanced by the introduction of a strong or noxious stimulus. This is not just the opposite of habituation since it depends on a strong stimulus, different from the one that elicits the reflex in question, but may act on presynaptic terminals within the reflex arc. In sensitisation, the response to a normal stimulus is greatly increased in amplitude and there is usually a decrease in response latency. For example, if an habituated *Aplysia* receives a noxious stimulus, such as a shock or blow to the head or tail, it will become sensitised to the next normal stimulation of the siphon and there will be a rapid withdrawal of the gill. At the cellular level, sensitisation in *Aplysia* is believed to be mediated by a set of facilitator neurones activated by noxious stimulation of the head or tail (Figure 3.13C). These neurones secrete the neurotransmitter, serotonin, direct application of which to the sensory neurones mimics sensitisation of the gill withdrawal response. This causes the second messenger, cyclic AMP, to act intracellularly to inactivate potassium channels in the presynaptic terminal membrane. Since potassium channels are responsible for repolarisation of the membrane following an action potential, the axon terminal remains depolarised for longer and causes calcium channels, whose opening is dependent on depolarisation (i.e. voltage-dependent calcium channels), to stay open for longer. This in turn allows more synaptic vesicles to bind to release sites on the presynaptic membrane and promotes the release of greater quantities of transmitter onto the motoneurone, resulting in facilitation of the psp.

Thus habituation results from the decrease in transmitter mobilisation which underlies synaptic depression, whilst sensitisation results from the increase in transmitter mobilisation which underlies synaptic facilitation.

3.8 Non-synaptic release of neurotransmitters

According to Vizi (1984), considerable evidence exists that neurones are able to release a variety of different substances from sites other than axon terminals. This clearly conflicts with

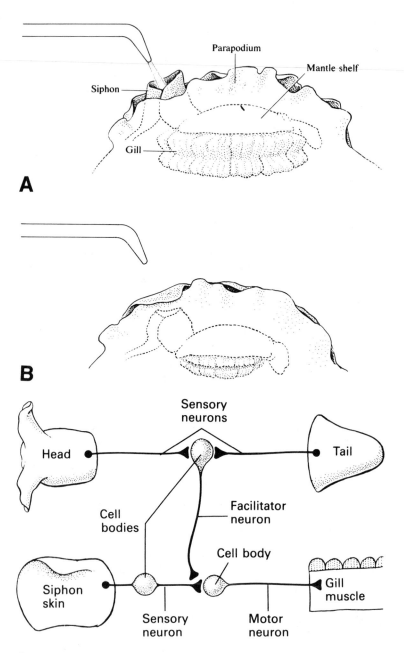

Parapodium

Mantle shelf

Siphon

Gill

A

B

Sensory
neurons

Head

Tail

Cell
bodies

Facilitator
neuron

Cell body

Siphon
skin

Gill
muscle

Sensory
neuron

Motor
neuron

C

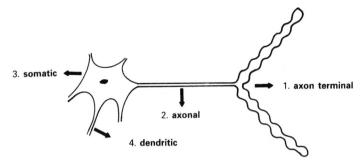

Fig. 3.14 Possible sites of transmitter release from a neurone: *conventional*, from the axon terminal (1); *unconventional*, from the axon (2), the soma (3) or the dendrites (4). (From Vizi, 1984.)

the classical view that neurotransmission occurs only at synapses and involves only a single secretory product for any given neurone. However, to take a well-known example, in neurones supplying smooth muscle contacts appear to be made at varicosities along the length of the axons and there is evidence that dendritic and somatic release may occur in other neurones (Figure 3.14). The release sites are often unspecialised and transmitter may act on neurones some distance away from the site of secretion. On the basis of these findings it would seem that, in addition to the mechanisms listed in the sections above, chemical communication in both the peripheral and central nervous systems is likely to be mediated:

(i) by non-synaptic axon terminals;
(ii) from axon terminals making synaptic contact but also acting on non-synaptic target cells;

Fig. 3.13 The defensive withdrawal reflex of *Aplysia*. A, The mantle cavity in the relaxed position, with the siphon and gill seen through the parapodia. B, the gill and siphon in the withdrawn position following a jet of seawater to the siphon. (From Kandel, 1976.) C, A simplified diagram of the neural circuits involved in the gill withdrawal reflex. Certain interneurones have been omitted for the sake of simplicity. (From Darnell *et al.*, 1986.)

(iii) from regions of the nerve cell other than the axon terminals, i.e. dendrites, soma and axon.

Future studies on the physiology of the nervous system will need to take these phenomena into account.

3.9 **Further reading**

(Other literature is listed in the compiled references at the end of the book.)

Bowman, W. C., Marshall, I. G., Gibb, A. J. and Harbone, A. J. (1988). Feedback control of transmitter release at the neuromuscular junction. *Trends in Pharmaceutical Sciences*, **9**, 16–20.

Eccles, J. C. (1957). *The Physiology of Nerve Cells*. Johns Hopkins Press, Baltimore.

Gray, E. G. (1977). Presynaptic microtubules, agranular reticulum and synaptic vesicles. In: *Synapses*, eds. G. A. Cottrell and P. N. R. Usherwood, pp. 6–18. Blackie, Glasgow.

Gray, E. G. (1978). Synaptic vesicles and microtubules in frog motor endplates. *Proceedings of the Royal Society of London*, B, **203**, 219–27.

Hille, H. (1984). *Ionic Channels and Excitable Membranes*. Sinauer, Sunderland, MA.

Israel, M., Dunant, Y. and Manaranche, R. (1979). The present status of the vesicle hypothesis. *Progress in Neurobiology*, **13**, 237–75.

Jones, D. G. (1981). *Neurones and Synapses. Studies in Biology, 135*. Edward Arnold, London.

Junge, D. (1981). *Nerve and Muscle Excitation*. Sinauer, Sunderland, MA.

Kandel, E. R. (1976). *Cellular Basis of Behavior*. Freeman, San Francisco.

Kandel, E. R. and Schwartz, J. H. (1982). Molecular biology of learning: modulation of transmitter release. *Science*, **218**, 433–43.

Kandel, E. R. and Schwartz, J. H. (1985). *Principles of Neural Science*, 2nd edition. Elsevier, New York.

Katz, B. (1969). *The Release of Neural Transmitter Substances.* Liverpool University Press, Liverpool.

Kuffler, S. W., Nicholls, J. G. and Martin, A. R. (1984). *From Neuron to Brain*, 2nd edition. Sinauer, Sunderland, MA.

Marchbanks, R. M. (1979). Role of storage vesicles in synaptic transmission. In: *Secretory Mechanisms, Symposium of the Society of Experimental Biology*, **33**, 251–76.

Osborne, N. N. (1983). *Dale's Principle and Communications between Neurones.* Pergamon Press, Oxford.

Shepherd, G. M. (1983). *Neurobiology.* Oxford University Press, New York.

Winlow, W. and McCrohan, C. R. (1987). *Growth and Plasticity of Neural Connections.* Manchester University Press, Manchester.

Young, S. H. and Chow, I. (1987). Quantal release of transmitter is not associated with channel opening on the neuronal membrane. *Science*, **238**, 1712–13.

Vizi, E. S. (1984). *Non-synaptic Interactions Between Neurons: Modulation of Neurochemical Transmission.* Wiley, Chichester.

4

Graded chemical transmission by non-spiking neurones

P. J. Simmons Department of Zoology, University of Newcastle-upon-Tyne

4.1 Introduction

Within nervous systems, great diversity is found in the mechanisms for transmitting and transforming information. Recently much attention has been paid to the increasing list of substances which are believed to be employed as neurotransmitters, and there is also considerable variation in the effects that transmitters have on the conductance of channels in postsynaptic membranes. There is also diversity in the operating characteristics of different synapses: in the relationship between changes in presynaptic and in postsynaptic potentials. For some time it has been realised that spikes (action potentials) are not required for synaptic transmission, and it is now established that many neurones normally operate without producing spikes. It was discovered in the 1950s that photoreceptors in the vertebrate retina do not usually spike, and signal changes in light intensity by graded changes in membrane potential. Since the mid 1970s, many examples have been described of interneurones which exert graded effects on the membrane potentials of postsynaptic neurones without the intervention of spikes. The division between 'spiking' and 'non-spiking' nerve cells is, however, not clear-cut. Three examples illustrate ways in which this division is blurred.

First, some recent studies show that non-spiking neurones may possess a complement of voltage-activated channels which is at least as rich as that of neurones which produce trains of spikes. In some neurones, voltage-activated channels can produce regenerative depolarisations which often generate small spikes of graded amplitude. Such neurones are apparently usually unable to produce trains of overshooting spikes.

Second, the amplitude of the postsynaptic potential at a synapse made by a spiking neurone can vary in a systematic manner. The best known example of this is at synapses between sensory neurones and gill withdrawal motoneurones in *Aplysia*, where changes in synaptic efficacy are thought to underly habituation and sensitisation of the gill withdrawal response (see also Chapter 3).

Third, in some neurones, the release of transmitter can be regulated both by spikes and by non-regenerative, graded changes in membrane potential. For example, in the small ganglion which controls stomach muscles in the spiny lobster, *Panulirus*, if spikes are blocked with pharmacological agents, regularly repeating and co-ordinated cycles of changes in membrane potential still occur. There is also evidence for local computations in neurones, mediated by graded potentials and not communicated to distant parts.

The purpose of this chapter is to describe the operating characteristics of synapses where the presynaptic neurone does not generate trains of spikes, and to relate the transfer characteristics of such synapses to the contexts in which they normally operate.

Much of our knowledge of the way in which transmitter release is controlled comes from two synapses: the neuromuscular junction in the frog, which is readily accessible, as it lies outside the central nervous system; and the squid giant synapse, where it is possible to vary the potential of the presynaptic potential over a wide range, and to measure the flow of ionic currents which mediate the release of transmitter. Both of these synapses act as relays, where a presynaptic spike is normally followed by a postsynaptic spike, and work on these synapses has often involved the use of pharmacological agents to block the spikes. Three findings are particularly important in any consideration of transmission at chemical synapses:

(i) Transmitter is released as small, definite-sized units, called quanta, each of which produces a discrete miniature postsynaptic potential. These are readily recorded from muscle fibres, but are usually difficult to detect in central neurones.

(ii) There is a graded relation between presynpatic potential and the release of transmitter. At the squid giant synapse, a sigmoid relation between changes in pre- and postsynaptic potential is revealed when spikes are blocked.

(iii) The release of transmitter is mediated by the entry of calcium into the presynaptic terminal, and the flow of calcium is directly proportional to the rate of transmitter release. Calcium enters the terminal through voltage-activated channels, and most of the delay in transmission is due to the time taken by these channels to open. For a further discussion of chemical synaptic transmission see Chapter 3.

4.2 Operating characteristics of a sensorimotor synapse in a crab

A study by Blight & Llinás (1980) on transmission between a sensory neurone and a motoneurone in the swimming crab, *Callinectes*, is the most detailed description to date of the operation of a synapse where the presynaptic neurone does not generate trains of spikes. Three stretch receptors monitor rotation of the hind leg relative to the thorax, and the study on synaptic transmission concerned the largest receptor, the 'T-fibre', which is embedded in a thin strand of receptor muscle parallel and close to the large muscle that promotes the leg. Stretching the receptor muscle produces a depolarising receptor potential in the T-fibre. Motoneurones of the promotor muscle are excited by the T-fibre, and so the synapse is part of a resistance reflex, similar to those mediated by muscle spindles in vertebrates. The promotor muscle is innervated by seven motoneurones, of which type I has the largest cell body. Postsynaptic potentials (psps) were usually recorded from the cell body because of its relatively large size and constant location. Arthropod motoneurone cell bodies are usually electrically inexcitable, and connected by a narrow neurite to the dendrites and axon. Psps probably decremented to 30–40% of their original amplitude as they travelled from the synapse to the cell body.

The likely site of synapses made between the T-fibre and promotor motoneurones is indicated by the region of closest apposition of membranes, seen in sections under the light microscope when the neurones are stained with cobalt salts or horse-radish peroxidase. Examination of the T-fibre in this region under the elecron microscope showed that it contains large numbers of synaptic vesicles concentrated near darkly-staining pre-synaptic densities. Postsynaptic elements were fine processes, probably originating from motoneurone dendrites.

The method employed by Blight & Llinás allowed them to vary presynaptic potential over a wide range (Figure 4.1A). The T-fibre was cut through close to the receptor muscle and the axon dissected free of others within the receptor nerve. The cut end was pulled through a narrow bath containing sucrose solution into a stimulating chamber. Because sucrose is a very poor con-ductor, when a potential difference was imposed between the stimulating and the main chambers, current flowed along the axon of the T-fibre and altered the transmembrane potential of the T-fibre.

The axon of the T-fibre is sometimes greater than $50\,\mu m$ in diameter, and this calibre is maintained into the CNS, past the region where the synapses with motoneurones are probably made. The axon is between 8 and 13 mm long. Correspondingly, the length constant of the T-fibre is large, so that the graded receptor potential is conducted with little decrement to the pre-synaptic zone. Although it is subject to some inaccuracy, the most straightforward way to derive the length constant is to insert two microelectrodes, separated by a known distance, into the axon, and to measure the decrement in amplitude of a potential as it travels towards the ganglion (Figure 4.1B).

The length constant can then be calculated as the distance separating the two electrode tips divided by the natural logarithm of the ratio of the potentials recorded at the two locations. Measurements from T-fibres indicate some considerable variation (3–60 mm) between different individual crabs in the value of the length constant, but it is always large enough for us to be sure that an electrode inserted anywhere in the axon within the CNS will record potentials very close to those which occur at the presynaptic site. Depolarising pulses of current can trigger regen-erative events in a T-fibre, as can be seen in Figure 4.1B, where there is a small spike.

The development of psps in a motoneurone, evoked by square

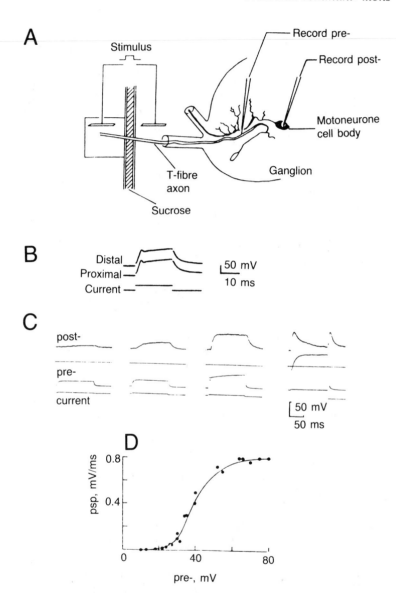

A

Stimulus

Record pre-

Record post-

Motoneurone
cell body

T-fibre
axon

Ganglion

Sucrose

B

Distal

Proximal

Current

50 mV

10 ms

C

post-

pre-

current

50 mV

50 ms

D

psp, mV/ms

0.8

0.4

0   40   80

pre-, mV

pulses of current of different intensities injected into a T-fibre, is shown in Figure 4.1C. Between current pulses, the inside of the T-fibre was held at −80 mV relative to the saline in the recording chamber, and the smallest postsynaptic response was detected when the T-fibre was depolarised by 10 mV from this holding potential. For larger presynaptic depolarising pulses, there was a synaptic latency of 1.3–1.4 ms. The transfer characteristics, which relate potential of a T-fibre to corresponding responses in a motoneurone, are plotted in Figure 4.1D. As at the squid giant synapse, the relation between presynaptic potential and post-synaptic response is an S-shaped curve. For presynaptic potentials up to 40 mV depolarised from the holding potential, the relation is exponential. In this range, for a tenfold increase in postsynaptic response, the T-fibre must be depolarised by 12.5 mV, a value which is close to the corresponding measurement made for the squid giant synapse. For more positive presynaptic potentials, the slope decreases and eventually reverses.

Fig. 4.1 Transmission at the synapse between the T-fibre and a leg promotor motoneurone in the swimming crab, *Callinectes*. A, Diagram summarising important features of the experimental preparation. Both the T-fibre and the motoneurone branch more extensively within the ganglion than is indicated here, and are drawn slightly separated from each other at the site of the synapse, for clarity. The motoneurone is black; the T-fibre is unshaded. Electrical stimuli were applied to the axon of the T-fibre by two silver electrodes; independent glass microelectrodes recorded pre- and postsynaptic potentials. The diagram is not drawn to scale. B, A square pulse of current was injected into the T-fibre, and the voltage recorded simultaneously at two points along it in order to measure its decrement. The distal electrode was 1 mm from the sucrose bath and the two recording electrodes were 0.65 mm apart. The length constant for this T-fibre was 10.5 mm. Notice: the T-fibre depolarised more rapidly than it repolarised to its original potential; the small spike-like response. C, Recordings of pre- and postsynaptic potentials when stimulating currents of different strengths were injected into a T-fibre. The second trace represents zero potential for the T-fibre. D, A graph relating presynaptic potential to the size of the psp when square pulses of current were injected into a T-fibre. The size of the psp is expressed as rate of depolarisation because this gives the most accurate measure of the release of transmitter. (B–D, taken from Blight & Llinás, 1980.)

At the squid giant synapse this is because the rate of transmitter release is reduced as the presynaptic potential approaches the equilibrium potential for calcium ions across the membrane, the 'suppression potential'. At the crab synapse, when a square pulse of current was injected to depolarise the T-fibre to 120 mV from the holding potential, there were two peaks in the postsynaptic response. The first occurred during the time taken for the T-fibre to depolarise and when it was fully depolarised transmission was suppressed. The second peak immediately followed the end of the pulse of current. The explanation for the second peak is that, when the presynaptic potential drops back to the holding level, the presynaptic calcium channels do not close immediately, so that calcium flows inward as the presynaptic potential moves away from the calcium equilibrium potential. The second peak in the psp shows that the decline which follows the first peak is not due to the depletion of transmitter.

A T-fibre can maintain a high level of transmitter output for long periods (Figure 4.2A). During a two-second-long pulse of depolarising current, the T-fibre remained depolarised by about 50 mV and the postsynaptic recording shows that transmitter was continually released. The psp amplitude was not constant, but showed two stages of decline, one occurring within 250 ms and the second lasting about 1 s.

There are a number of possible explanations for the two stages of decline, including desensitisation of postsynaptic receptors, inactivation of calcium currents in the presynaptic terminal, or a decline in the store of transmitter available for release. Blight and Llinás favoured the last explanation, and suggest that the final, sustained psp level represents the rate at which transmitter can be turned over metabolically.

There is evidence, based upon an analysis of the quantal release of transmitter from receptor cells in the ear of fish, that stimulation by sound leads to a rapid decline in the amount of transmitter available for release. It has been proposed that increasing sound intensities can activate greater numbers of discrete stores of transmitter. At the crab synapse, following a long depolarisation, recovery of the full ability to transmit takes 1.5 s.

An idea of the amount of activity which can probably occur at the presynaptic terminal during prolonged transmission can be

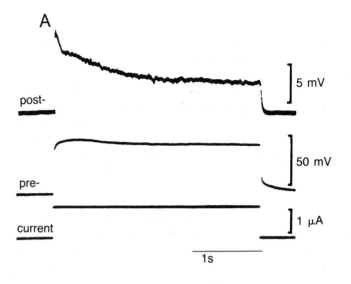

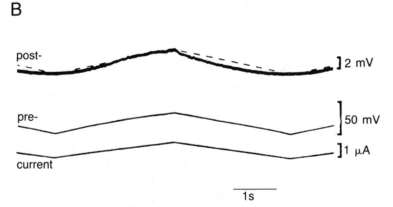

Fig. 4.2   Changes in psp amplitude during long-lasting current stimuli injected into a crab T-fibre. A, During a 2 s-long pulse of depolarising current the T-fibre depolarised to an almost constant level. The psp showed a rapid initial stage of in decline, followed by a slower decline to a level which was sustained through the second half of the current pulse. B, Slow ramps of depolarising and hyperpolarising current were injected into the T-fibre. The presynaptic potential follows the current closely but the psp is distorted. In particular, at the start of the hyperpolarising phase of the stimulus, the motoneurone potential changed more rapidly than that of the T-fibre. (From Blight & Llinás, 1980.)

gained from the following estimate, made by Blight and Llinás, of the turnover of membrane. From the postsynaptic region of motoneurones, they recorded some small epsps 150–200 μV in amplitude. If this represents the psp mediated by one quantum of transmitter, the rate of quantum release to generate a psp of 30 mV would be 30 000 per second. This is similar to the rate of vesicle discharge following the arrival of a spike at motoneurone terminals at the frog neuromuscular junction. If each quantum corresponds to one vesicle, which discharges by fusion with the presynaptic membrane, then, in maintaining a high rate of transmission to all seven promotor motoneurones, 588 μm² would be added to the presynaptic membrane of a T-fibre each second. The surface area of the presynaptic zone is 10 000–20 000 μm².

Before the study by Blight and Llinás, it was known from work by Bush and colleagues (see Roberts & Bush, 1981) on a smaller crab, *Carcinus*, that small changes in T-fibre potential are correlated with quite large changes in the frequency of spikes in promotor motoneurones. Examination of the transfer characteristics of the synapse shows one mechanism behind this, as well as other ways in which the operation of the synapse is related to its role in mediating a postural reflex. In an intact crab, the dendrites of the receptor are probably usually under some tension, both as a result of the angle of the joint which the receptor spans, and of activity of motoneurones of the receptor muscle. As a result of the tension, the T-fibre would be depolarised above the threshold for transmitter release, and this has two important consequences. First, because transmitter would be released continually, the synapse can convey information about decreases as well as increases in tension. Second, the slope of the curve relating T-fibre potential to psp size is greatest when the T-fibre is depolarised by 20–30 mV from the threshold for transmitter release (Figure 4.1D). This means that to maximise the sensitivity of the rate of transmitter release to small changes in presynaptic potential, the membrane potential of T-fibre should be held in this range.

In the control loop of which this synapse forms a part, there are a number of stages at which delays occur, including those for synaptic transmission and for the development of muscular tension. The way in which the rate of transmission has an initial peak, and then declines top a steady plateau level (Figure 4.2A) shows that the gain of the synapse depends on the recent history of T-fibre membrane potential. This can be interpreted as compensating for these delays. Following a rapid stretch to the receptor muscle, the gain of the synapse will be high, but when the T-fibre hyperpolarises, following a relaxation of the receptor muscle, gain of the synapse will be less. This will help to bring about a rapid decline in the amplitude of the psp in the motoneurone, and consequently in the rate of spikes it produces. Figure 4.2B shows that the gain of the synapse is different during depolarising and hyperpolarising ramps of current injected into the T-fibre. Such relatively slow ramps are probably more likely to occur in the T-fibre of an intact, moving crab than are rapid, square-shaped changes in potential.

One of the problems associated with employing graded potentials rather than spikes for transmission along an axon is that it limits the speed at which membrane potential can change. This is because in order to transmit a potential with little decrement in amplitude, the axon must have a relatively high value for transmembrane resistance, r_m. The length constant λ is given by $\lambda = r_m/r_i$, where r_i is the longitudinal resistance of the axoplasm. However the time constant of the membrane, τ, is also related to r_m: $\tau = r_m.C_m$, where C_m is the capacitance of the membrane. The ability of the T-fibre to produce regenerative depolarising potentials is a way of compensating for the smoothing of potentials and delays in their transmission, which would occur if the membrane were purely passive, and is important in speeding up the reflex response to increased stretch of the receptor.

The axon of the T-fibre contains a number of different voltage-activated channels. The flow of current through these channels has been studied by Mirolli (1983), in voltage clamp experiments on isolated lengths of T-fibre axon taken from the crab *Portunus*. There is an initial fast inward current, carried by sodium ions, similar to the current which underlies the depolarising phase of the action potential in the squid giant axon. However, the T-fibre does not generate trains of spikes, and the regenerative response is of graded amplitude, rarely overshooting zero potential. One reason for this may be that the density of sodium channels is low. Another is that the sodium current is followed very quickly by an outward current carried by potassium ions. Both these currents are activated within 1 ms, and are inactivated at potentials more positive than -50 mV: the potassium current responsible for the hyperpolarising phase of the action potential in the squid giant synapse is activated more slowly than this, and does not inactivate. In the T-fibre, there is also a second, relatively slow and long-lasting, potassium current. A likely function for this is to limit the amplitude of depolarisation caused by large-amplitude stretches, so that the receptor can code for a wide range of strengths of stretch, without compromising the ability to discriminate between small stretches of different strengths.

4.3 Non-spiking interneurones in the thoracic ganglia of insects

There is good evidence that non-spiking interneurones are important in the control of postural and rhythmical activity in insects and crustacea. The most extensive study is by Burrows and Siegler (1978) on non-spiking interneurones which synapse with motoneurones that control movements of the hind legs of a locust. Each hind leg is controlled by about 50 motoneurones, which have relatively large cell bodies, $30-90$ μm across. The locations of these cell bodies are fairly constant from animal to animal, so that an intracellular recording can be made in different experiments from a chosen motoneurone. By recording from a motoneurone and simultaneously from an interneurone, it was established that many of the interneurones which synapse with the leg motoneurones operate without spiking. The morphologies of two non-spiking interneurones, both of which excited the single slow motoneurone of the muscle that extends a hind leg, are shown in Figure 4.3A. Morphological features which all these non-spiking interneurones share are: that they are local to the metathoracic ganglion, although some arborise on both sides of it; they have no process to which the term 'axon' can reasonably be applied; and that they branch extensively within the neuropil, where their processes intermingle with those of motoneurones and other interneurones. Non-spiking interneurones which have similar physiological effects can have quite different shapes. Although the relative proportion of spiking to non-spiking interneurones is not known, representatives of both groups are frequently encountered by an electrode probing the neuropil, and there have been estimated to be about 1000 local interneurones within this ganglion.

A non-spiking interneurone mediates smoothly graded amplitudes of psp upon neurones it connects with. This is shown by using an electrode to inject pulses of current of different strengths into an interneurone, while recording from a postsynaptic motoneurone (Figure 4.3B) or interneurone. Because the same electrode is used both to measure membrane potential and to inject current, accurate measurement of the change in potential that a pulse of current causes in the interneurone cannot be made.

Injection of depolarising current into the interneurone caused the motoneurone to hyperpolarise, so the synapse was inhibitory. Hyperpolarising current injected into the interneurone current caused the motoneurone to depolarise, which shows that the interneurone was releasing transmitter tonically between current pulses. The graded effect that an interneurone can have on motoneurone potential is converted into a graded effect upon the frequency of spikes in the motoneurone and, in turn, into a graded effect on muscle tension.

A single interneurone can make excitatory connections with some motoneurones, and inhibitory connections with others. An interneurone typically controls motoneurones of more than one muscle, so that the interneurones make connections which can control movements involving several joints. Non-spiking interneurones also make connections with each other. These connections are always inhibitory and one-way, which is appropriate for different interneurones to be employed in co-ordinating different patterns of muscular activity.

Is it the normal mode of operation for these interneurones to exert graded effects on motoneurones without using spikes? This question is important because it is possible that the neurones are damaged during an experiment, which might inactivate the spike-generating mechanism. No spikes have ever been reported to have been produced by injection of current into them, and a number of careful controls against effects of damage were made. Other local interneurones within the same ganglion, and recorded using the same techniques, do produce trains of spikes.

Quite small amounts of current injected into an interneurone can mediate psps. This suggests that small potential changes, of

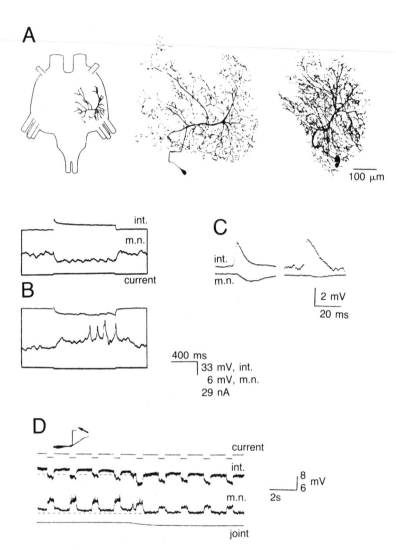

Fig. 4.3 Non-spiking interneurones which connect with leg motoneurones in the metathoracic ganglion of a locust. A, The morphologies
of two interneurones, both of which made excitatory connections with
the slow extensor tibiae motoneurone. The drawing on the left shows the
outline of the ganglion and the main processes of the neurone which is
drawn in more detail in the centre. The two interneurones were stained
by intracellular injection of cobalt ions, and later intensified by deposi-

the order of $1-2$ mV, might affect the rate of release of transmitter. Evidence that this is so comes from recordings shown in Figure 4.3C. The interneurone made a short-latency inhibitory connection with a motoneurone of the muscle that flexes the hind leg. When the leg was forcibly flexed, a resistance reflex was activated, in which discrete epsps just over 2 mV in amplitude were recorded from the interneurone. In turn, each epsp was followed by a discrete ipsp in the motoneurone. That the interneurone was part of the pathway mediating these ipsps was shown by injecting hyperpolarising current into it, which reduced the ipsp amplitude.

The effects that non-spiking interneurones mediate on motoneurones differ according to the behavioural context. In Figure 4.3D, an interneurone was repeatedly injected with pulses of current of identical strength. When the leg was extended, each pulse of current caused the motoneurone to spike, presumably by reducing the release from the interneurone of a transmitter which inhibited the motoneurone. When the leg was flexed to a right-

---

tion of silver onto the cobalt. They are viewed dorsally. B, A depolarising and a hyperpolarising pulse of current injected into an interneurone each caused a change in membrane potential in the fast flexor tibiae motoneurone. One microelectrode was inserted into the interneurone in a process in the neuropil, and was employed both for recording from and injecting current into the interneurone. Although the current caused a deflection in the recording from the interneurone, this is not a reliable measure of the change in membrane potential of the interneurone. C, Epsps in this interneurone mediated ipsps in a flexor tibiae motoneurone. The epsps were produced when the leg was held flexed. In the record on the right, the interneurone was hyperpolarised by injecting 3 nA of hyperpolarising current into it. This hyperpolarising current reduced the size of the ipsps, although the amplitude of the epsps was slightly increased. The recordings are averages of 32 individual psps. D, During this recording from a non-spiking interneurone and a flexor tibiae motoneurone the angle of the knee joint is altered. Regularly repeated pulses of -3 nA current were injected into the interneurone, which made an inhibitory connection with the motoneurone. Half-way through the record, the knee joint was flexed from an extended to a half-flexed angle, and there the change in postsynaptic potential which each current pulse caused was altered. (A, Taken from Siegler & Burrows, 1979; B, from Burrows & Siegler, 1978; C, from Burrows, 1979; and D, from Siegler, 1981.)

angle, both the neurones hyperpolarised slightly, and the pulses of current did not evoke spikes in the motoneurone. So sensory neurones, which monitor the angle and movements of the leg, can alter the effectiveness of the connection. There are a number of probable pathways for this effect, involving synaptic inputs to one or both neurones.

4.4 Graded interactions between visual neurones

In the vertebrate retina, the first three layers of cells (receptors, horizontal cells and bipolar cells) do not normally spike, and neither do some types of cell in the next layer, the amacrine cells. This means that most synaptic interactions in the retina must occur by way of graded interactions, where the release of transmitter is controlled in a continuous manner by membrane potential. The first demonstrations of graded interactions were indirect, either using pharmacological means to block transmission, or recording extracellularly from ganglion cell axons while injecting current into receptors. More recently, in retinas of fish and amphibians, pairs of interconnected cells have been penetrated with microelectrodes. The recordings in Figure 4.4A and B were made from a slice of the retina of a salamander, *Ambystoma*, and electrodes were inserted simultaneously into a rod photoreceptor and a bipolar cell. In vertebrates light causes photoreceptors to hyperpolarise. Injection of hyperpolarising current into the receptor also caused the bipolar cell to depolarise (Figure 4.4A). This shows that the rod made an inhibitory connection with this bipolar cell and also that, in the dark, the rod was continually releasing transmitter.

The vertebrate retina contains cone as well as rod photoreceptors, and the effects of the two receptors on the bipolar cell are distinguished in Figure 4.4B. Following a bright flash, a cone repolarises rapidly to its initial dark potential, whereas voltage in a rod and in a bipolar cell (recorded simultaneously) declined slowly and were linearly correlated during the decline. In the intact retina, each bipolar cell may receive inputs from as many as 500 rods, and this high degree of convergence helps to maximise sensitivity in conditions of low illumination.

Because light hyperpolarises a vertebrate photoreceptor, the effect of illumination is to reduce the rate of transmitter release from the receptor. This means that, under most normal conditions of illumination, the receptor will be continually releasing transmitter; both increases or decreases in illumination can be converted into changes in the rate of transmitter release. Another result is that the synapse can make use of the most sensitive region of the curve relating input to output. Most invertebrate photoreceptors depolarise upon illumination and there is good evidence that, in the dark, their membrane potentials are also depolarised from the threshold for transmitter release. In the compound eye of the fly, very small signals can be transmitted from photoreceptors to second-order neurones called large monopolar cells (lmcs). Because the receptors and lmcs are small and numerous, it is not feasible to record from synaptically-linked pairs. However, the transfer of signals between receptors and lmcs can be studied by recording from them separately, but under identical conditions of illumination. The signal caused by absorption of a single photon of light can be transmitted from a photoreceptor to an lmc (Figure 4.4C). Each photon causes a discrete depolarising bump in the photoreceptor. The corresponding bumps in an lmc are hyperpolarising, so the synapse is inhibitory, and they are three times as large, so the synapse has a gain, in the dark, of -3. Considering the exponential relation between membrane potential and transmitter release, it is very likely that, in the dark, the receptor constantly releases transmitter. The bumps are six times as frequent in an lmc as in a receptor, which correlates with detailed anatomical studies showing that six photoreceptors converge on each lmc, each receptor making about 220 anatomically distinct synapses. This convergence helps to maximise both sensitivity to low illumination, and the signal-to-noise ratio.

In addition to inversion and amplification, there are time-dependent changes as signals pass from photoreceptors to second-order neurones in arthropods. In Figure 4.4D simultaneous recordings were made from a photoreceptor and a large second-order neurone (L-neurone) of the simple eye, or ocellus, of a dragonfly. The responses of the L-neurone to increases and to decreases in light intensity are more phasic than those of the photoreceptor. An important consequence is that the L-neurone does not signal background light intensity but rather variations around it, as can be seen by comparing the two recordings. In

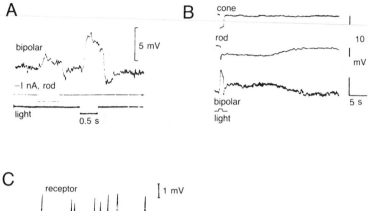

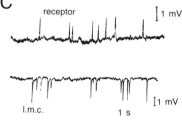

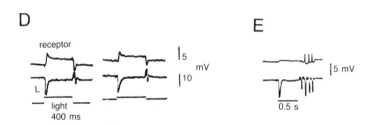

Fig. 4.4   Graded transmission between visual neurones. A, Electrodes were inserted simultaneously into a rod photoreceptor and a bipolar cell in a thin section taken from the retina of a tiger salamander. Both the injection of hyperpolarising current into the rod, and a 0.5 s-long flash of light caused the bipolar cell to depolarise. B, Recordings of responses to a bright flash of light from cells in a thin slice of a salamander retina. The bipolar cell and rod were recorded simultaneously, and injection of current into the rod (as in Fig. 4.4A) showed that it connected with the bipolar cell. The recording from the cone photoreceptor was made from the same preparation 15 min later. C, Recordings of the responses to single photons of light in a photoreceptor and a large monopolar cell (lmc) in the compound eye of a fly. Note the difference in voltage calibrations. During the recording from the lmc, the intensity of the

both, the intensity of the light flash was the same, but the recording on the left was made in the dark whereas the recording on the right was made during continual background illumination. The amplitude of the depolarising response by an L-neurone to 'light off' is boosted by regenerative properties of its membrane; L-neurones often produce single spikes of graded amplitude. The mechanism for boosting the response to 'light on' relative to the response to sustained illumination is probably that the rate of transmitter release declines during a constant presynaptic depolarising potential. Decrement in transmission is seen in Figure 4.4E where, following a flash of light, a photoreceptor generated a short train of spikes. This is an unusual response caused by injury to the receptor. Each spike mediated an ipsp in the L-neurone, and the decline in ipsp amplitude from spike to spike is clear. This record shows psps mediated by potential change in a single photoreceptor: in ocelli, hundreds of recetors converge onto a single L-neurone.

4.5 Voltage-activated currents in non-spiking neurones

Analysis of the conductance properties of a number of non-spiking neurones has shown that they are far from being cables of passive membrane – they contain a quota of voltage-active channels as great as that found in spiking neurones. The vetebrate photoreceptor, for example, has at least five voltage-activated currents, and will produce trains of large spikes if bathed in saline containing TEA, which blocks potassium channels, and high cal-

---

stimulating light was less than during the recording from the photoreceptor. D, Recordings made simultaneously from a photoreceptor and from a large second-order neurone (L-neurone) of a dragonfly ocellus. The intensity of the flash of light was the same in both records but there was no background illumination in the left recording, whereas the flash was superimposed on a constant background light in the recording on the right. E, Simultaneous recordings from a photoreceptor and L-neurone in an ocellus of another dragonfly. The photoreceptor had been damaged by the electrode, and produced a train of spikes at the end of a pulse of light. Each spike mediated an ipsp in the L-neurone. (A, B, Taken from Wu, 1985; C, from Dubs *et al.*, 1981; D, E; from Simmons, 1982.)

cium (Figure 4.5A). Because calcium enters neurones through voltage-activated channels at presynaptic sites, then all neurones must contain at least some voltage-activated channels. Usually calcium currents are very small and unlikely to generate large spikes. Some non-spiking neurones, including the crab T-fibre and ocellar L-neurone, have regenerative sodium channels which speed up the rate at which the neurone can depolarise. In order to limit depolarising regenerative responses, a number of mechanisms are possible, including setting the resting potential to a level at which sodium currents are partially or completely inactivated, and employing potassium currents. Some amacrine cells of the vertebrate retina normally only produce single spikes in response to a depolarising stimulus (Figure 4.5B). The mechanism for this involves a potassium current which acts to clamp the potential of the neurone at a level which prevents reactivation of the sodium current.

L-neurones of insect ocelli also produce single spikes. One function for these spikes has been found by studying transmission at inhibitory connections which some L-neurones make with each other. Here separate electrodes can be employed to inject current presynaptically and record presynaptic potential, while psps are also measured (Figure 4.5C). Ipsp amplitude varies with the amplitude of the presynaptic spike, but the duration of an ipsp is severely limited so that, even if a long-lasting pulse of current is injected presynaptically, the ipsp starts to decline 7 ms after its start. Because the decrement in transmission is so rapid, the presynaptic neurone must depolarise rapidly in order to mediate any appreciable psp. Following an ipsp, a connection recovers its ability to transmit over about 1 s. Recovery occurs even if the presynaptic neurone is held depolarised during this time. This makes it unlikely that depletion of transmitter stores is responsible for the rapid decrement in transmission. A more likely mechanism is that calcium channels at the presynaptic sites inactivate.

Some neurones appear to be able to switch between a spiking and a non-spiking state. Ocellar L-neurones of the bee provide an example (Figure 4.5D). This switching demands further investigation: what is its mechanism and what are the effects on the release of transmitter from the neurone?

4.6 Local computations in neurones

One of the major difficulties in understanding how networks of neurones work is that a neurone cannot necessarily be regarded as a single functional entity. Signals do not always spread to all parts of a neurone, and parts of a neurone can participate independently of each other in local computations. Anatomical studies of the distribution of synapses show that input and output synapses sometimes occur close together, providing a structural framework for local interactions. A good example is shown in Figure 4.6, where a small part of an identified, spiking interneurone in the locust was painstakingly reconstructed from serial sections. The concept of local computations goes hand-in-hand with the realisation that small graded potentials can regulate the release of transmitter, since non-involvement of spikes enables physiological independence between different parts of a neurone. Theoretical studies on the ways in which potentials travel within neurones reveal how anatomy can affect independence of different parts. Such studies have been made on non-spiking interneurones in the locust, and on 'starburst' amacrine cells of the vertebrate retina. They have shown that, if a potential travels passively from a small branch to a larger one, it will decline greatly in amplitude. On the other hand, a synapse made onto a small branch will generate a larger psp than if it were made onto a larger branch. Fine branches interlink regions of wider branches in the starburst cells, and provide a mechanism for isolating different regions from each other. So far it is not known whether input synapses to non-spiking neurones occur largely on small branches.

4.7 Perspective: Variations in the control of transmitter release

One feature common to all synapses where the appropriate measurements have been made is that there is an S-shaped transfer curve which relates pre- and postsynaptic potentials. Synapses differ: in the part of the curve over which they normally operate; in the maximum slope of the curve, or the 'gain' of the synapse; and in changes in the relation between pre- and postsynaptic potentials with time.

At synapses where the presynaptic neurone produces trains of

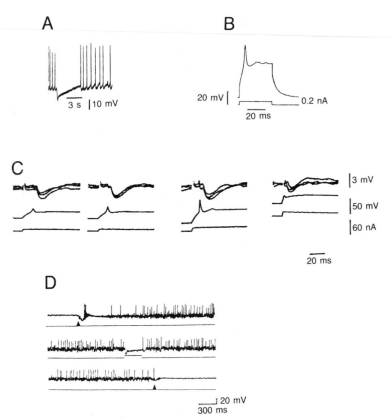

Fig. 4.5   Spikes in neurones which normally do not produce trains of spikes. A, Spikes recorded from a rod of a toad retina which was perfused with saline containing TEA and twice normal calcium concentration. During a flash of light, the receptor hyperpolarised and spiking stopped. B, Recording from an amacrine cell in the retina of a tiger salamander. A pulse of 0.2 nA current caused it to fire a single spike, which was followed by a sustained depolarisation. C, Transmission at an inhibitory connection made between to L-neurones of a locust ocellus. Separate electrodes were used to inject current into and record membrane potential from the presynaptic neurone. Current is monitored on the bottom trace, presynaptic potential on the middle trace, and ipsps on the top trace. In the first three records, the presynaptic neurone was initially hyperpolarised from its normal resting potential. Each record shows three ipsps superimposed. D, Intracellular recording from an ocellar L-neurone in a bee. When a background light was switched on (first arrow) the neurone started producing spikes, and continued until

overshooting spikes, the whole of the transfer curve is used. The squid giant synapse is an example of this kind of synapse. During the peak of a spike, presynaptic potential exceeds the calcium equilibrium potential and, in fact, most transmitter is released during the repolarising phase of the spike. Because the whole of the transfer curve is used, then small variations in spike ampli- tude, due perhaps to fluctuations in temperature or in osmotic pressure, will not affect psp size; this might be important for a synapse which functions as a reliable relay of spikes. Where the presynaptic neurone does not spike, the synapse can use the shape of the transfer curve to convey smoothly graded potentials. If the presynaptic neurone has a resting potential depolarised from the threshold for transmitter release, then both polarities of change in potential can be transmitted, and the synapse can convey small changes in presynaptic potential because it will use the steepest part of the transfer curve. The slope of the steepest part of this curve is the maximum gain of the synapse. The squid giant synapse and crab sensorimotor synapses have very similar maximum gains, but there is probably considerable variation in maximum gain between different synapses. The synapse which links photoreceptors to lmcs in the fly compound eye, for ex- ample, where a high gain enables detection of very small light stimuli.

Some synapses can maintain high rates of transmitter release for prolonged periods while, at others, the rate of release de- clines during a prolonged presynaptic depolarisation. Vertebrate photoreceptors release transmitter continually in the dark and must be able to maintain a high rate of replenishment of trans- mitter. At the other extreme, at inhibitory connections between some insect ocellar L-neurones, transmission is curtailed after a few milliseconds and production of ipsps is dependent on the regenerative properties of the presynaptic neurone which enable it to depolarise rapidly before decrement of transmission starts.

the background light was switched off (second arrow). During the period of background illumination, additional light directed at the ocellus (step in light monitor trace) hyperpolarised the neurone and inhibited the spikes. (A, Taken from Fain *et al.*, 1977; B, from Barnes & Werblin, 1986; C, from Simmons, 1985; D, from Milde, 1981.)

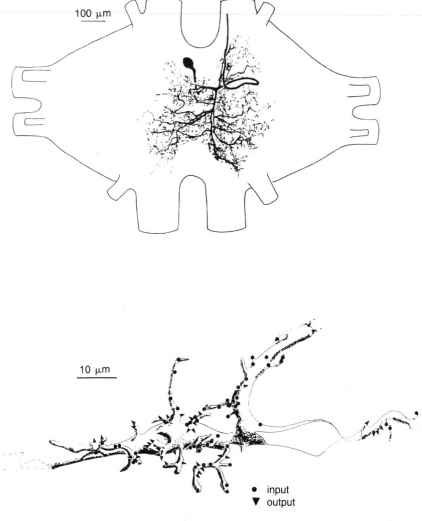

Fig. 4.6 Input and output synapses on a small region of an identified interneurone in the locust. A drawing of the interneurone viewed dorsally within the second thoracic ganglion is shown in the upper part of the figure. The interneurone has been stained by cobalt and later intensified with silver. A characteristic morphological feature of this interneurone is the loop which is made by the axon within this ganglion. The axon travels at least as far as the first thoracic ganglion, and the interneurone

Decrement of transmission is, at some synapses, clearly a mechanism which enables them function efficiently. At the crab sensorimotor synapse, for instance, it enables rapid decrease in potential in a motoneurone when the T-fibre relaxes; at synapses made by photoreceptors, it enables second-order neurones to maintain high sensitivity to changes in illumination, while the photoreceptors operate over a very wide range of background intensities.

The mechanisms which give synapses different properties are largely unknown. Recently it has been clear that there is considerable diversity in the types of calcium channels found in neurones. Some, for example, can remain open for long periods; others inactivate rapidly. Synapses at which the presynaptic calcium channels inactivate rapidly would show rapid decrement in transmission. A major experimental challenge is to correlate the properties of calcium channels in the presynaptic terminals of non-spiking neurones to the operating characteristics of their synapses.

4.8 Further reading

(Other literature is listed in the compiled references at the end of the book.)

Bader, C. R., Bertrand, D. & Schwartz, E. A. (1982). 'Voltage-activated and calcium-activated currents in solitary rod inner segments from the salamander retina', in *Journal of Physiology*, **331**, 253–84. (Describes a number of distinct conductances in a vertebrate photoreceptor.)

Barnes, S. & Werblin, F. (1986). Gated currents generate single

---

is excited by mechanical stimuli to the wings and feet. Below is a drawing of a three-dimensional reconstruction of a 16 μm-long section of the interneurone, in the region of the branch of two major processes. The reconstruction was made from a series of adjacent thin sections, which were examined under an electron microscope to reveal details of synaptic structure. Input and output synapses occur intermingled on this short region of the neurone. (Taken from Watson & Burrows, 1983; drawings kindly provided by A. H. D. Watson.)

spike activity in amacrine cells of the tiger salamander retina. *Proceedings of the National Academy of Sciences USA*, **83**, 1509–12.

Blight, A. R. & Llinás, R. R. (1980). The non-impulsive stretch-receptor complex of the crab: a study of depolarization-release coupling at a tonic sensorimotor synapse. *Philosophical Transactions of the Royal Society of London, Series B*, **290**, 219–76.

Burrows, M. (1979). Synaptic potentials effect the release of transmitter from locust nonspiking interneurons. *Science*, **204**, 81–3.

Burrows, M. & Siegler, M. V. S. (1978). Graded synaptic transmission between interneurones and motor neurones in the metathoracic ganglion of the locust. *Journal of Physiology*, (*London*), **285**, 231–55. (This paper describes the graded nature of transmission between local non-spiking interneurones and motoneurones, and details the evidence that these interneurones normally operate without using spikes.)

Calvin, W. H. & Graubard, K. (1979). Styles of Neuronal Computation. *The Neurosciences. Fourth Study Program*, eds. F. O. Schmitt and F. G. Worden, pp. 513–24. Massachusetts Institute of Technology Press, Cambridge MA. (A thought-provoking account of integrative processes in neurones, which emphasises the diversity of mechanisms which occur in neurones. This volume also contains other articles of relevance to the topic of synaptic transmission by non-spiking neurones.)

Dubs, A., Laughlin, S. B. & Srinivasan, M. V. (1981). Single photon signals in fly photoreceptors and first order interneurons at behavioural threshold. *Journal of Physiology*, **317**, 317–34.

Fain, G. L., Quandt, F. N. & Gerschenfeldt, H. M. (1977). Calcium-dependent regenerative responses in rodents. *Nature*, **269**, 707–10.

Llinás, R. R. (1982). Calcium in synaptic transmission, *Scientific American*, **247**, 38–47. (An account of the involvement of calcium in regulating the release of transmitter at the giant synapse of the squid.)

Milde, J. (1981). Graded potentials and action potentials in the large ocellular interneurons of the bee. *Journal of Comparative Physiology A*, **143**, 427–34.

Miller, R. J. (1987). Multiple calcium channels and neuronal function, *Science*, **235**, 46–52.

Miller, R. F. & Bloomfield, S. A. (1983). Electroanatomy of a unique amacrine cell in the rabbit retina, *Proceedings of the National Academy of Sciences, USA*, **80**, 3069–73. (About the 'starburst' amacrine cell.)

Mirolli, M. (1983). Inward and outward currents in isolated dendrites of crustacean coxal receptors, *Cellular and Molecular Neurobiology*, **3**, 355–70.

Roberts, A. & Bush, B. M. H. (eds.) (1981). *Society for Experimental Biology Seminar Series, No. 6*. Cambridge University Press, Cambridge. (A comprehensive collection of papers outlining work on non-spiking neurones up to 1980, which provides a useful background to many of the topics described here.)

Siegler, M. V. S. (1981). Postural changes alter the synaptic interactions between nonspiking interneurons and neurons of the locust. *Journal of Neurophysiology*, **46**, 296–309.

Siegler, M. V. S. (1984). Local interneurones and local interactions in arthropods, *Journal of Experimental Biology*, **112**, 253–81. (A useful summary of the anatomy and physiology of local interneurones in invertebrates.)

Siegler, M. V. S. & Burrows, M. (1979). The morphology of nonspiking local interneurones in the metathoracic ganglion of the locust. *Journal of Comparative Neurology*, **183**, 121–48.

Simmons, P. J. (1982). The operation of connexions between photoreceptors and large second-order neurones in dragonfly ocelli. *Journal of Comparative Physiology A*, **149**, 389–98.

Simmons, P. J. (1985). Postsynaptic potentials of limited duration in visual neurones of a locust, *Journal of Experimental Biology*, **117**, 193–213. (This paper concerns the short-lasting nature of transmission at some synapses of an insect ocellus.)

Watson, A. H. D. & Burrows, M. (1983). The morphology, ultrastructure and distribution of synapses on an intersegmental interneurone in the locust. *Journal of Comparative Neurology*, **214**, 154–69.

Wu, S. M. (1985). Synaptic transmission from rods to bipolar cells in the tiger salamander retina, *Proceedings of the National Academy of Sciences, USA*, **82**, 3944–7.

5

Peptide neurotransmitters

G. J. Dockray MRC Secretory Control Research Group, University of Liverpool

5.1 Introduction

Little more than a decade ago it seemed likely that there were relatively few chemical neurotransmitters. The transmitters recognised at that time (acetylcholine, noradrenaline, dopamine, glycine, glutamate, serotonin, GABA) appeared sufficient to account for the known range of synaptic responses. It was, however, already well known that biologically active peptides could be produced by neurones. The earliest of these to be characterised were the neurohormones of the hypothalamo-hypophyseal tract, i.e. oxytocin and vasopressin, and from the late 1960s onwards a series of releasing factors had also been isolated from hypothalamus: the first was thyrotropin releasing hormone (TRH), which was soon followed by luteinizing hormone releasing hormone (LHRH) and the growth hormone inhibitory factor, somatostatin. Initially, the releasing factors were thought to be more or less exclusively concerned with regulation of the anterior pituitary. It soon became clear, however, that these as well as other peptides, many of them first found in the gut, were distributed widely throughout the central and peripheral nervous systems, and that they were capable of exerting potent effects on many different neurones and other cells. These observations have given rise to the idea that peptides might have neurotransmitter or neuromodulator functions.

Recent progress in the characterisation of peptide transmitters and modulators can be attributed to several factors. In particular, modern microchemical methods have allowed the minute quantities of peptides found in nervous tissue to be isolated and fully characterised with relative ease; similarly molecular biological methods have allowed the cloning and sequencing of the genes encoding neuropeptides. In addition, the ready availability of immunochemical methods of detection has made possible both the quantitative estimation of neuropeptides in tissue extracts and their cellular localisation. Finally, developments in peptide chemistry, notably solid phase synthesis, have facilitated the production of synthetic peptides on a large scale. As a consequence biological studies no longer depend on the availability of natural peptides which all too often can be obtained from tissue extracts only in small amounts.

At the cellular level there are many similarities in the mechanism of action of neuropeptides and classical transmitters. However, peptides can act over distances and times that are greater than is often thought to be the case for the classical transmitters; there are also important differences in the way that peptides and classical transmitters are handled by neurones. For these reasons, therefore, special considerations apply in studying the physiology of neurones that act through the release of peptides, i.e. *peptidergic neurones*.

5.2 **Peptide families and their distribution**

Many neuropeptides can be grouped into families on the basis of their structural relationships (Table 5.1). In some instances the different peptides in a family have a common biosynthetic origin, in other instances they share a common evolutionary origin. The latter can usually be attributed to duplication of an ancestral gene and divergence of the daughter genes through point mutation. Different family members may have widely different functions and distributions. One of the largest and most diverse families consists of glucagon, gastric inhibitory peptide (GIP), vasoactive intestinal peptide (VIP), peptide histidine isoleucine amide (PHI), growth hormone releasing factor (GRF) and secretin. Three are produced in endocrine cells of the gut or pancreas (secretin, glucagon and GIP) and have digestive or metabolic hormonal functions, and three are neuropeptides (VIP, PHI, GRF). The occurrence of peptides with related structures is of importance in several regards. The different members of a family

Table 5.1   *Family groupings of the main mammalian neuropeptides*

VIP-Glucagon:
  VIP, PHI
  Glucagon
  GRF
  Secretin
  GIP
	Hypothalamo-hypophyseal peptides:
	  Oxytocin
	  Vasopressin
	
	Neurotensin:
	  Neurotensin
	  Neuromedin N

Tachykinins:
  Substance P, Substance K
  Neurokinin B
	Cholecystokinin:
	  CCK
	  Gastrin

Opioids:
  Enkephalin pentapeptides
  β Endorphin
  Dynorphin
	Others
	  Somatostatin
	  TRH
	  LHRH

Pancreatic polypeptide:
  Neuropeptide Y
  Peptide YY
  Pancreatic polypeptide
	Insulin
	  CGRP
	  Bradykinin
	  Angiotensin
	  Insulin

Bombesins:
  Gastrin-releasing peptide
  Neuromedin B
	Corticotropin releasing factor
	  Neuromedin U

Note: The families are based on structural similarities between peptides. All the families have at least one member that has been isolated and sequenced from brain; in many families there are members that are not neuronal in origin but all the peptides shown are thought to have regulatory (hormonal, paracrine, etc.) functions. See text for definition of abbreviations.

may interact with the same receptors and so have similar biological actions. This can offer special insight into the nature of the peptide sequence that is functionally important, but it also means that special care is needed in interpreting the physiological significance of the responses evoked by a particular peptide. Similarly, antibodies raised to one peptide may cross react with structurally related substances. In using immunochemical methods to identify, measure and localise peptides, then, it is important to take steps to ensure the specificity of the reaction. For example antibodies to the shared C-terminus of gastrin and cholecystokinin (CCK) may cross-react with both peptides, but antibodies to the unshared regions allow these peptides to be localised and measured separately (Table 5.2).

Table 5.2 *Sequences and distribution of the gastrin-CCK group of peptides*

	Sequences	Distribution
Vertebrate Peptides		
Pig CCK8	-Asp-Tyr-Met-Gly-Trp-Met-Asp-Phe-NH$_2$	CNS, PNS, intestinal endocrine cells
Pig gastrin	-Glu-Ala-Tyr-Gly-Trp-Met-Asp-Phe-NH$_2$	Pituitary, gastric endocrine cells
Caerulein	-Asp-Tyr-Thr-Gly-Trp-Met-Asp-Phe-NH$_2$	Amphibian skin.
Chicken gastrin	Phe-Tyr-Pro-Asp-Trp-Met-Asp-Phe-NH$_2$	Chicken pyloric antrum.
Invertebrate Peptides		
Leucosulfakinin I	-Glu-Asp-Tyr-Gly-His-Met-Arg-Phe-NH$_2$	Cockroach CNS
Leucosulfakinin II	-Asp-Asp-Tyr-Gly-His-Met-Arg-Phe-NH$_2$	Cockroach CNS

Note: The main representative of the family in mammalian brain is CCK8. Only the C-terminal octapeptides are shown; outside this sequence the structural similarities are not impressive. In gut endocrine cells there are N-terminally extended forms of CCK8 with 33, 39 and 58 residues. Porcine gastrin occurs naturally as peptides of 17 and 34 residues extended at the N-terminus. Caerulein is a decapeptide, chicken gastrin is a 36-residue peptide and leucosulfokinins I and II are undeca and decapeptides respectively. In all these peptides the tyrosine can occur in the sulphated form. In CCK8 there is virtually complete sulphation. Note that the leucosulfakinins have some similarities to mammalian gastrin, and also to the molluscan neuropeptide Phe-Met-Arg-Phe-NH$_2$.

5.2.1 *Phylogenetic aspects*

Neurones that produce and secrete peptides are found in the
nervous systems of all major animal groups, including the primitive nerve net of the coelenterates. Many neuropeptides are
apparently well conserved. There is, for instance, immunochemical evidence for peptides resembling mammalian CCK,
the opioids, and the tachykinins, in a variety of invertebrate
neurones. In addition, elaborate systems of other peptide transmitters have recently been found in molluscan and arthropod
nervous systems (Kaldany *et al.*, 1985; O'Shea & Schaffer, 1985).
In *Aplysia*, several of the genes encoding neuropeptides have
been cloned and sequenced. These genes are expressed in neurones that may also contain classical transmitters. Together they
are responsible for the control of behaviours involved in egg lay-
ing and feeding. The molluscan nervous system offers several
advantages for this type of work, because neurones can be repro-
ducibly identified in different animals and are often very large. It
would not be surprising, however, to find that in other species
similar peptides were involved in the integrative control of different neuronal functions.

5.2.2 *Brain–gut and other relationships*

The genes encoding many neuropeptides are often expressed in
several types of cell. A good example of this is the production
of peptides, e.g. CCK (Table 5.2), somatostain, substance P,
neurotensin, ACTH/β-endorphin, both in the endocrine cells of
the mammalian gut, pancreas or pituitary, and in central or
peripheral neurones (Dockray, 1987). It seems likely that where
the same or related peptides are produced in different systems,
they have separate physiological roles. In general, peptides in the
circulation that act as hormones do not penetrate the blood–brain
barrier, and so cannot gain access to the CNS, except through
regions where the barrier is 'leaky'. This helps to maintain specificity of action when the same substance has both hormonal and
neurotransmitter functions.

5.2.3 *Mapping neuropeptides*

Physiological studies of neuropeptides depend, in the first instance, on a knowledge of their distribution. Two complementary types of immunochemical method provide the necessary
information. Quantitative information on tissue concentration

can be obtained by radioimmunoassay of tissue extracts. The identity of the immunoreactive material in tissue extracts needs to be verified by chromatographic separation and by the use of a variety of antibodies that differ in their specificity. This type of approach does not, however, give information on the precise cellular origins of the peptide. Immunocytochemistry provides information on localisation at the cellular or subcellular levels. As mentioned above, however, antibodies can react with a variety of structurally related peptides and care is therefore needed in interpreting immunohistochemical findings. Many of the peptides listed in Table 5.1 have been mapped in detail in the rat nervous system (Palkovits, 1984). Several generalisations can be made about neuropeptide distribution:

(i) the major mammalian neuropeptides each have a distinctive pattern of distribution in the central and peripheral nervous systems;

(ii) particular peptides are not exclusively localised to a single system, generally they occur in many different systems – for example early studies on substance P first revealed it in over 30 groups of nerve cells;

(iii) peptides occur in neurones together with classical transmitters and together with other structurally unrelated peptides. Thus the idea that nerve cells act through a single transmitter substance (sometimes mistakenly called Dale's principle) is now no longer tenable;

(iv) some parts of the nervous system are rich in neuropeptides, e.g. the hypothalamus, amygdala, substantia gelatinosa of the spinal cord, and the nerve plexuses of the gut, whereas others are generally poor in neuropeptides, e.g. the cerebellum and thalamus;

(v) peptides may be useful markers of subsets of nerve cells. Subpopulations of retinal amacrine cells, and of GABA neurones in the cerebral cortex, may be identified on the basis of their neuropeptide content.

5.3 Criteria for chemical neurotransmission

In trying to determine whether or not a substance acts as a chemical neurotransmitter, a variety of criteria are usually applied. These are: (i) that the substance should be present within a neurone, and synthesised there; (ii) that it should be released by depolarisation through a calcium-dependent mechanism; (iii) that the effect of stimulating the neurone is mimicked by exogenous application of the substance in all circumstances including, for example in the presence of the appropriate antagonists; and (iv) that there should be mechanisms for inactivation or termination of the response, which can include re-uptake of the transmitter into nerve terminals. These criteria can be said to have been satisfied, at least in outline, for many peptides. However, they date from a time before the discovery of peptide transmitters and do not take account of several distinctive and important features of peptidergic neurones. In particular, an understanding of biosynthetic mechanisms is of special importance, and depends in turn on elucidating the gene sequence encoding a peptide and determining the routes of mRNA and post-translational processing. Since peptides frequently occur in the same cells as classical transmitters, it is also necessary to establish: (i) the pattern of coexistence in particular neurones; and (ii) the relative rates of secretion of multiple transmitters from that neurone.

5.3.1 *Organisation of peptidergic neurones*
There are at least three important ways in which the mechanisms of synthesis and turnover of neuropeptides differ from those of classical transmitters (Figure 5.1). First, the capacity for protein, and therefore peptide synthesis is limited to the cell soma. Neuropeptides are therefore made first in the cell body and packaged there into granules or vesicles that are transported intra-axonally to the terminal regions prior to release. In contrast, the synthesis of classical transmitters, like acetylcholine or noradrenaline, can take place at the nerve terminal providing, of course, that the appropriate enzymes have been delivered there. Second, there is little or no evidence to suggest the occurrence of re-uptake mechanisms for neuropeptides. Following release, therefore, a peptide may either interact with a receptor on a target cell membrane, or be degraded, or diffuse away. In all events, there is only a single opportunity to exert a biological effect. In contrast, classical transmitters, or their immediate biosynthetic precursors, may be taken up again by the nerve terminal and recycled; this is in itself one way of terminating

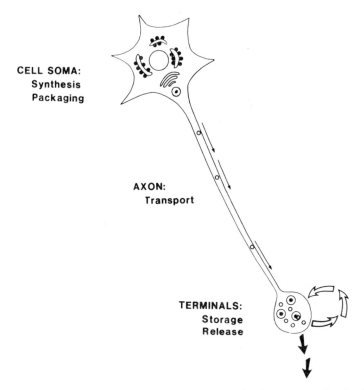

CELL SOMA:
Synthesis
Packaging

AXON:
Transport

TERMINALS:
Storage
Release

Fig. 5.1 Schematic representation of a peptidergic neurone. Synthesis and packaging of peptides into granules is limited to the cell soma; processing of large precursor peptides (cleavage of the precursor chain, and modification of individual residues, e.g. amidation, sulphation, glycosylation, phosphorylation) occurs in the Golgi region and in immature granules. Secretory granules are transported intraxonally to nerve terminals. At the terminals there is storage and release. There are no known mechanisms for re-uptake or re-utilisation of peptides following their release (➡). In contrast, classical transmitters may be made in nerve terminals and there are mechanisms for re-uptake of the transmitter or their immediate precursors (⇨). Note that the same neurone may release both peptide and chemical transmitters.

action, but it also offers the capacity to re-use or conserve transmitter. Third, the biosynthesis of neuropeptides is complex in that it virtually always includes the production of several different peptides. There is seldom a unique product following expression of a particular gene. In addition to the main active product generated by expression of a neuropeptide gene, there may also be inactive peptides, and peptides that have biological actions quite different to those of the primary active peptide or that show relatively subtle differences in activity.

5.4 Biosynthesis

The pathways of biosynthesis of neuropeptides have attracted considerable attention and are of great physiological importance (Eipper *et al.*, 1986; Lynch & Snyder, 1986). The cellular mechanisms of neuropeptide synthesis are the same as those of other secretory peptides. Genes are transcribed into mRNA, which in turn is translated into the peptide precursor that is then sequested into granules and processed to the final peptide products. The general rule is that small secretory peptides are synthesised initially as large precursor molecules.

The nucleotide base sequences of the genes encoding many neuropeptides have now been elucidated. Knowing the gene sequence does not, however, provide unequivocal information on the identity of the final peptide product. This is because at both of two different levels in the biosynthetic pathway there are mechanisms that influence the identity of the products: namely alternative pathways of mRNA processing, and alternative pathways of post-translational processing. The DNA sequence of a particular gene virtually always consists of sections that are transcribed into mRNA (exons) separated by intervening sequences (introns) that are not represented in mRNA species. During mRNA transcription the splicing of exons may proceed in a similar way in all cells expressing a particular gene. But there are cases where there is cell-to-cell variability at this stage so that one or more exons are sometimes spliced out of the final mRNA. Two good examples are provided by peptides that occur in primary sensory neurones: calcitonin gene related peptide (CGRP) and the tachykinins, substance P and substance K. When the gene encoding the hormone calcitonin is expressed in thyroid 'C' cells, the initial transcript is spliced to give an mRNA that encodes calcitonin but not CGRP. In certain neurones including some primary afferents, however, transcription of the same gene yields an mRNA in which the calcitonin-coding region is omitted and instead an additional sequence encoding a quite distinct peptide, CGRP, is incorporated. Similarly, the mRNA for the important tachykinin, substance P, exists in at least two forms. Both of them encode substance P, but one also encodes a second tachykinin, substance K, while in the other the portion which corresponds to substance K is omitted (Figure 5.2 top).

After translation of mRNA, the precursor peptide is further modified or processed. Peptide precursors almost invariably have an initial N-terminal signal sequence of about 20 amino acid residues that identifies the peptide as being destined for secretion, and which directs its passage across the rough endoplasmic reticulum (Figure 5.2). Soon thereafter the signal sequence is removed and it is seldom possible to find or measure this part of the precursor. Further biosynthetic processing occurs in the Golgi region and in immature secretory granules and takes the form of cleavage of the peptide chain and modification to individual aminoacid residues. Cleavage often occurs at pairs of basic residues, or at individual arginine residues, and is thought to depend on the action of two types of enzyme, one resembling trypsin in specificity, the other carboxypeptidase B. The products of cleavage generated at this stage are stored and secreted in parallel. Further modifications to them include C-terminal amidation, which is a feature common to about half of all neuropeptides, sulphation of tyrosines, glycosylation, N-terminal acylation, and phosphorylation. Each of these processing steps can exert profound effects on biological activity. The intact precursor frequently has little or no activity, and cleavage to liberate a free C- or N-terminus of the peptide product is generally needed for biological activity; similarly C-terminal amidation is essential for full activity of many peptides, as is sulphation, e.g. CCK8, while N-terminal acylation may abolish it, e.g. β-endorphin.

The precursors of some neuropeptides are relatively simple insofar as they contain a single copy of a biologically active sequence, e.g. CCK (Figure 5.2). Multiple forms of active peptides may nevertheless be produced from these precursors by variable patterns of cleavage around the active segment. Other precursors may be more complex and consist of:

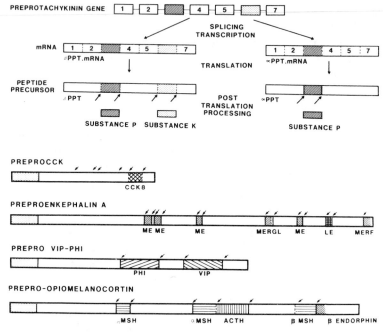

Fig. 5.2 (Top panel) Schematic representation of the biosynthetic pathway of substance P and substance K. There are seven exons in the DNA
sequence, one of which (6) encodes substance K. Two possible mRNA
species are generated: in one (β PPT) all the exons are represented,
in the other (α PPT) the substance K encoding region is omitted. Of the
two precursors that can be generated, one is able therefore to give rise
to both substance P and substance K, the other only to substance P.
(Bottom panel) Schematic representation of the organisation of the
precursors for CCK, the enkephalin pentapeptides (ME, Met enkephalin; LE, Leu-enkephalin), VIP-PHI and prepropiomelanocortin (MSH,
melanocyte stimulating hormone, ACTH, adrenocorticotrophin). Each
has an N-terminal signal sequence. Cleavage at the arrows generates
biologically active products (allowing for C-terminal amidation where
appropriate). Note, however, that there are cell-specific patterns of
cleavage of each of these precursors. In the case of CCK for example,
CCK8 is the main product in brain, but in gut endocrine cells N-
terminally extended forms of 33, 39 or 58 residues occur in high concentrations as well (the latter are generated by cleavage at points to the
N-terminus of the CCK8 sequence, see arrows).

(i) multiple copies of the same sequence, e.g. pentapeptide sequence of Met-enkephalin – which occurs six times in its precursor;

(ii) multiple copies of different but structurally related peptides, e.g. VIP–PHI which are derived from a common precursor;

(iii) copies of several distinct active peptides, e.g. ACTH, β-endorphin and the melanocyte stimulating hormones (MSHs).

Many examples are known of cell-specific pathways of post-translational processing. This means that different cells process the same precursor in different ways to yield distinct peptide products. In the case of CCK, the predominant processing pathway in brain yields the octapeptide (CCK8), but in gut endocrine cells CCK8 occurs together with larger N-terminally extended forms of 33, 39 or 58 residues. These forms have similar affinities for CCK receptors. But only the largest forms pass through the liver and so these are particularly suited for hormonal functions. In the CNS there are no such constraints on the delivery of active forms of CCK to their receptors. A further well studied example of cell specific processing is the ACTH–β-endorphin precursor, propiomelanocortin, which is processed by different pathways in cells of the pars intermedia, pars distalis, and arcuate nucleus.

5.5 Secretion and metabolism

Release by exocytosis is common to all protein secretory cells, including peptidergic neurones. Release studies are conveniently performed *in vitro* using either small slices of brain, or synapto-somal preparations (pinched-off nerve endings). This type of study allows more careful control of the external medium than can be obtained *in vivo*. The release of all neuropeptides has an absolute requirement for calcium and can be evoked by depolar-isation, for example by increasing extracellular K^+ concentrations (Figure 5.3). It is also possible to modify secretion with other transmitters. One early example was the demonstration that opioids would depress substance P release from trigeminal slices (Iversen *et al.*, 1980). Recent approaches to the study of release *in vivo*, have involved push–pull cannulae or perfusion through

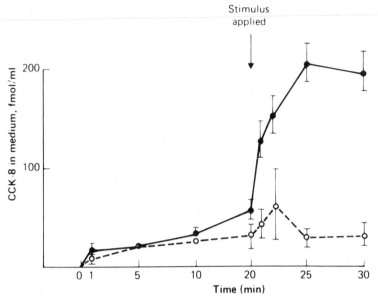

Fig. 5.3 Release of immunoreactive CCK from cortical slices of rat brain. The slices were incubated in Krebs–bicarbonate solution and CCK in the medium was measured by radioimmunoassay. The stimulus, depolarisation by 52.2 mmol L^{-1} K^+, was applied to both preparations. In one ($\bullet$) calcium 2.5 mmol L^{-1} was also present, in the other ($\circ$) it was omitted. Note calcium-dependent release on depolarisation. (Taken from Dodd *et al.* 1980.)

dialysis fibres inserted into the brain. The great advantage of these methods is that secretion can be studied *in situ*, although the quantities of peptide released are frequently very small.

   Proteolytic enzymes that degrade neuropeptides are widely distributed. Much of the available information on the metabolism of neuropeptides is based on studies of peptide degradation by different fractions of brain homogenates. The results provide a rational basis for the development of peptide analogues that are resistant to degradation, and they also allow the development of inhibitors of enzyme action that can be used *in vivo*. Some of the most intensively studied peptides in this regard are the opioid pentapeptides, Leu and Met enkephalin (Tyr[1]-Gly[2]-Gly[3]-Phe[4]-

Met^5 or Leu^5). There are several enzymes in the brain that degrade these peptides; of special importance are those that cleave the peptide bonds between Tyr^1-Gly^2 and Gly^3-Phe^4. The enzyme involved in the latter cleavage has been studied by several research groups – some of whom called it enkephalinase. It is, however, the same as an enzyme that was first found in the kidney and termed endopeptidase 24.11; it degrades many different peptides by cleaving to the N-terminal side of hydrophobic residues. Inhibitors of this enzyme, e.g. thiorphan, are able to potentiate the action of opioid peptides because they block degradation and so increase peptide concentrations *in vivo*. The enzyme(s) cleaving the Tyr-Gly bond appears to account for a high proportion of the total enkephalin degradation. Cleavage at this site is sensitive to substitutions in the Gly^2 position of the peptide chain. Thus replacing glycine in position two with D-alanine produces an analogue that is resistant to degradation but is still biologically active; such analogues are better able to reach receptors (and so are active in lower doses) and they also produce longer lasting responses than the native pentapeptides. Other substitutions also increase resistance to degradation but it should be remembered that they can also change affinity for different types of opioid receptors.

5.6 Receptors and antagonists

Like other water-soluble intercellular messenger molecules, peptides exert their effects by first binding to cell-surface receptors, and thereafter activating one of a relatively small group of transduction systems. Notable amongst these is the regulation of cyclases and control of intracellular cyclic nucleotide concentrations, or stimulation of the hydrolysis of phosphatidyl inositol and the consequent liberation of the two intracellular mediators – diacylglycerol, which activates protein kinase C, and inositol trisphosphate which liberates calcium from endoplasmic reticulum. The coupling of receptors to second messenger systems depends on G proteins. But neither these, nor the second messengers themselves are specific for peptides or any other single class of ligand. One of the important actions of intracellular signalling systems is to regulate ion channel opening or closing. Whether or not peptide receptors are also able to gate ion channels directly, analogous to the nicotinic acetylcholine receptor-channel is not yet certain, although there is no objection to it in principle.

A common feature of many transmitter systems is the occurrence of more than one receptor type; the multiple receptors for acetylcholine, noradrenaline, and dopamine are all familiar examples. There are also multiple receptor types for many peptides. In the first instance these can be identified by comparing the rank order of potency of various analogues in different test systems, e.g. bioassays, binding studies, second messenger responses; they can also be characterised by examining the action of different antagonists on a range of agonists. Two examples are worth citing. In the case of the opioids, there are at least three receptor types: mu, kappa, and delta (Kosterlitz & Paterson, 1985). Considerable effort has been devoted to establishing the likely endogenous ligands for the different types of opioid receptor. The dynorphins are often considered likely ligands for kappa receptors, the enkephalin pentapeptides for delta receptors, while β-endorphin may act at both mu and delta. The distribution of mu and delta receptors generally matches that of the enkephalins, but the match of kappa receptors and their potential ligands is less impressive. A good example of the significance of the distribution of receptor types is provided by CCK. There are at least two major types of receptor for CCK. One of these, which can be called the peripheral receptor, occurs on pancreatic acinar cells, gall bladder muscle, myenteric neurones, and probably vagal fibres; these receptors show high affinity for CCK and at least 1000-fold lower affinity for the related peptide gastrin. These receptors are of course exposed both to gastrin and CCK in the blood, and their specificity ensures that they are activated only by CCK. A similar type of receptor may occur in certain discrete regions of the brain; but the predominant CCK binding site in brain, which can be called the central receptor, shows only about 10–50 times lower affinity for gastrin compared with CCK. The CNS receptors are not normally exposed to gastrin and their relatively higher affinity for gastrin does not therefore compromise the specificity of their response to CCK.

Physiological studies of peptidergic systems depend on antagonists and these are still difficult to find. In the case of substance

P and LHRH, useful analogues with antagonist activity have been developed by substituting residues (often D-amino acids) in the primary peptide structures. Antagonists that are themselves peptides may be valuable for many experimental studies, but for therapeutic applications they suffer from the disadvantage that they are rapidly degraded, do not readily penetrate the blood–brain barrier, and are often ineffective when given orally. These problems may be overcome to varying degrees by developing non-peptide antagonists. The opioid antagonist, naloxone, is a good example that has been known for many years, but in general it has been difficult to develop non-peptide antagonists for neuropeptides. However, remarkable progress has been made recently with substances that antagonise the peripheral type of CCK receptor. Several different types of CCK antagonist have been recognised for some time, but since they have low affinity they have not been suitable for *in vivo* work. While screening fermentation broths for possible CCK antagonists, a research group at Merck Sharp and Dohme Laboratories discovered a metabolite of the fungus *Aspergillus* that has weak CCK antagonist properties and which they named asperlicin. There are similarities in structure between asperlicin and the benzodiazepines, and on this basis a range of benzodiazepine analogues were screened for CCK antagonist properties. This led to the discovery of an excellent antagonist for peripheral CCK receptors, L364,718. This compound does not interact with the 'benzodiazepine–receptor'. It is orally active and doses of a few μg produce effective blockade of peripheral CCK receptors for several hours in the rat.

5.7 Peptidergic systems

An impressive variety of behavioural effects have been described in mammals in response to neuropeptides administered either peripherally (intravenous or interperitoneally) or centrally (into the cerebral ventricles or directly into discrete areas of brain). Some striking examples are the analgesic effects of opioid peptides, the actions of CCK in inhibiting food intake, the effects of ACTH and vasopressin fragments on memory and learning, and the effects of LHRH on reproductive behaviour (see Krieger *et al.*, 1983). Care is needed in interpreting the physiological significance of findings based on peripheral administration of neuropeptides. It is now clear, for instance, that the actions of peripherally administered peptides may be exerted outside the CNS. Thus, in the rat, CCK probably inhibits feeding by acting on vagal afferent nerve endings and this effect is independent of the central neurotransmitter function of the peptide. In the vertebrates some of the best examples of peptidergic neuroeffector transmission are found not in the CNS but in the periphery, where it is possible to study in detail the connections and actions of peptidergic neurones.

5.7.1 *Primary afferents and peptides*

Peptides are well represented in primary afferent nerve fibres. Substance P was one of the earliest of these peptides to be studied. Long before it was isolated and characterised, Lembeck had noted higher concentrations of substance P bioactivity in dorsal, compared with ventral, spinal roots and had raised the idea that this substance might be a transmitter in afferent neurones. It is now clear that substance P is indeed synthesised in dorsal-root ganglion cells, particularly small diameter cells. The same neurones also synthesise CGRP (although there are probably further CGRP-containing primary afferents that do not contain substance P); other peptides (somatostatin, VIP, bombesin) may also be produced in certain primary afferents. The peptides synthesised in dorsal-root ganglia cells are transported to central terminals in the dorsal horn, where they are released and participate in the central transmission of information following $A\delta$ and C fibre stimulation. Interestingly, however, the major proportion of the material synthesised in these neurones is directed not centrally but to peripheral terminals. Axon collaterals of primary afferents that contain substance P and CGRP are found around blood vessels in the skin and joints, and in the gut they occur around myenteric ganglion cells and submucosal blood vessels, they also make contact with ganglion cells as they pass through the sympathetic prevertebral ganglia. Stimulation of primary afferents results not just in the conduction of action potentials towards the CNS, but also in the release of substance P and CGRP at peripheral terminals. It has been known for very many years that antidromic stimulation of afferents produces a vasodilator response in the skin and an increase in local blood flow. Both substance P and CGRP have vasodilator actions and are good candidates for this effect. In addition substance P increases capillary permeability and produces plasma extravasation. These effects are in part direct, but they also involve release of histamine from mast cells which augments the increase in blood flow and capillary permeability.

5.7.2 *Autonomic neuroeffector transmission*

The combined use of cholinergic and adrenergic antagonists over the last 20 years has produced many examples of so-called 'non-adrenergic, non-cholinergic transmission' in the autonomic nervous system. Purines were one of the first groups of substances considered as candidate transmitters for these effects; in addition, though, there is now good evidence that peptides account for many types of autonomic non-adrenergic non-cholinergic transmission (Dockray, 1987).

A clearcut case is the effect of parasympathetic stimulation on salivery gland function. Electrical stimulation of the chorda tympani increases both the flow of saliva and blood flow in the submaxillary gland. Atropine blocks the flow of saliva indicating cholinergic-muscarinic transmission, but the increase in blood flow remains. Postganglionic parasympathetic fibres to the salivary gland contain both acetylcholine and VIP. By radioimmunoassay of the venous effluent during electrical stimulation, two groups of workers, one in Cambridge, the other in Stockholm, have been able to show release of VIP. One of the actions of VIP is to induce vasodilatation. The atropine-resistant vasodilation can therefore be attributed to the effect of VIP. This is not an isolated example: there is evidence of a similar type to suggest that VIP mediates the effect of vagal stimulation on the flow of pancreatic juice in some species, and on the inhibition of gastric motility in the presence of atropine. Other probable peptidergic effects in the gut include substance P mediation of non-cholinergic smooth muscle contraction in the peristaltic reflex, and the release of gastrin by the bombesin-like substance, gastrin releasing peptide.

5.7.3 *Ganglionic transmission*

The study of ganglionic transmission has provided excellent examples of peptidergic effects. One such example is the transmission from preganglionic fibres to ganglion cells in ninth and tenth paravertebral sympathetic ganglia in the bullfrog (Jan & Jan, 1982). There are two types of ganglion cells, large B cells and small C cells. Stimulation of preganglionic fibres produces four types of response: a fast nicotinic-cholinergic excitatory post-synaptic potential (epsp), a slow muscarinic epsp and inhibitory postsynaptic potential (ipsp), and a non-cholinergic late slow epsp. In B cells the fast epsp is seen following stimulation of 3rd, 4th and 5th spinal nerves, but the slow epsp is seen only with the 7th and 8th spinal nerve stimulation. Stimulation of the latter nerves also produces similar synaptic responses in C cells. In the presence of total cholinergic blockade the late slow epsp persists. Several lines of evidence suggest that LHRH mediates this effect (Figure 5.4): (i) it is mimicked by application of LHRH, and its agonists; (ii) it is blocked by LHRH antagonists; (iii) there is immunochemical data to suggest the presence of LHRH-like material in preganglionic fibres and its release by stimulation of preganglionic nerves. The localisation of the peptide revealed by immunohistochemistry is striking, however, because it appears that LHRH-like immunoreactivity is not found in terminals located on the large B cells of the ganglia; instead it occurs in association with terminals around smaller C cells. Evidently, LHRH diffuses from terminals around C cells to the B cells. This illustration provides direct evidence, then, for the view that pep-

---

Fig. 5.4   (Top panel) A, the late slow epsp (N) in bullfrog sympathetic ganglion B cells in response to nerve stimulation, and application of LHRH (L). B, After incubation with the LHRH antagonist (D-pGlu[1], D-Phe[2], D-Trp[2,6]) LHRH, $10^{-5}\,\mathrm{mol\,L^{-1}}$ M, both late slow epsp and responses to LHRH were abolished. At the side, the fast epsp was not affected by the antagonist. (Bottom panel) Organisation of the innervation of bullfrog sympathetic ganglia. LHRH immunoreactive nerve terminals surround the smaller C-cells but not B cells. Both cells have a cholinergic innervation and both show the LHRH-induced late slow epsp. Evidently LHRH must diffuse to the B cells to produce this effect. (Both panels reproduced from Jan & Jan, 1982.)

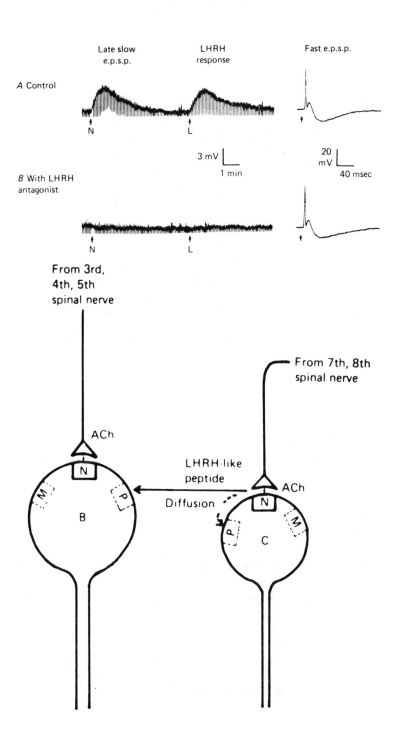

tides are able to act over greater distances and times than classical transmitters.

There is not, at present, evidence for a role of LHRH in mammalian sympathetic ganglion transmission. There is, however, good evidence for the involvement of substance P in transmission in the prevertebral ganglia (Otsuka & Konishi, 1983). Primary visceral afferents pass through the prevertebral ganglia. Approximately 50% of the spinal afferents to the upper gastrointestinal tract contain substance P (Dockray & Sharkey, 1986). Axon collaterals of these fibres terminate on some prevertebral sympathetic ganglia cells. Stimulation of the fibres to the guinea-pig inferior mesenteric ganglion produces a slow non-cholinergic epsp that is mimicked by substance P. Two further lines of evidence suggest that SP is responsible for the late epsp in this ganglion. First, substance P antagonists the action of both substance P and the non-cholinergic epsp. Secondly, the neurotoxin, capsaicin, which first stimulates and then inhibits small diameter primary afferent neurones including those containing substance P, is able to block the slow epsp.

5.8 **Further reading**

(Other literature is listed in the compiled references at the end of the book.)

Dockray, G. J. (1987). Physiology of enteric neuropeptides. In: *Physiology of the Gastrointesinal Tract (2nd edn)*. Ed. L. R. Johnson pp. 41–66. Rasen Press, New York.

Dockray, G. J. & Sharkey, K. A. (1986). Neurochemistry of visceral afferent neurones. *Progress in Brain Research*, **67**, 133–48.

Dodd, P. R., Edwardson, J. A. & Dockray, B. J. (1980). The depolarization-induced release of cholecystokinin C-terminal octapeptide (CCK. 8) from rat synaptosomes and brain slices. *Regulatory Peptides*, **1**, 17–29.

Eipper, B. A, Mains R. E. & Herbert, E. (1986). Peptides in the nervous system. *Trends in Neurosciences*, **9**, 463–68.

Iversen, L. L., Lee, C. M., Gilbert, R. F., Hunt, S. & Emson, P.

E. (1980). Regulation of neuropeptide release. *Proceedings of the Royal Society of London, B*, **210**, 91–111.

Jan, L. Y. & Jan, Y. N. (1982). Peptidergic transmission of sympathetic ganglia of the frog. *Journal of Physiology*, **327**, 219–46.

Kaldany, R-R., Nambu, J. R. & Scheller, R. H. (1985). Neuropeptides in identified *Aplysia* neurons. *Annual Review of Neuroscience*, **8**, 431–55.

Kosterlitz, H. W. & Paterson, S. J. (1985). Types of opioid receptors: relation to antinociception. *Philosophical Transactions of the Royal Society of London, B*, **308**, 291–7.

Krieger, D. T., Brownstein, M. J. & Martin, J. B. (eds.) (1983). *Brain Peptides*. Wiley Interscience, New York.

Lynch, D. R. & Snyder, S. H. (1986). Neuropeptides: Multiple molecular forms, metabolic pathways, and receptors. *Annual Review of Biochemistry*, **55**, 773–39.

O'Shea, M. & Schaffer, M. (1985). Neuropeptide function: The invertebrate contribution. *Annual Review of Neuroscience*, **8**, 171–98.

Otsuka, M. & Konishi, S. (1983). Substance P – the first peptide neurotransmitter? *Trends in Neurosciences*, **6**, 317–25.

Palkovits, M. (1984). Distribution of neuropeptides in the central nervous system: A review of biochemical mapping studies. *Progress in Neurobiology*, **23**, 151–89.

Receptor-mediated secondary messengers in the nervous system

A. B. Tobin and **N. N. Osborne** Nuffield Laboratory of Ophthalmology, Oxford

6.1 Introduction

Many hormones and neurotransmitters regulate neuronal activity by the generation of secondary messengers. The role of these secondary messengers is to act as a transduction medium through which extracellular communication between cells results in a physiological response. The generation of probably the most widely studied secondary messenger, cyclic $3',5'$-adenosine monophosphate (cAMP), was first demonstrated in the brain by Sutherland and coworkers (Robinson *et al.*, 1971). Cyclic AMP has been shown to regulate a variety of neuronal functions mainly by the activation of specific phosphorylation reactions (Nestler & Greengard, 1984). Less well understood, but of undoubted importance in the nervous system is another cyclic nucleotide secondary messenger, cyclic $3',5'$-guanosine monophosphate (cGMP). The number of neurotransmitters utilising cGMP as a secondary messenger is far smaller than that for cAMP, nevertheless it has been implicated in the regulation of many neuronal activities, in particular cerebellum Purkinje cell function (Schlichter *et al.*, 1978) and phototransduction in the vertebrate photoreceptor outer segments (Cook *et al.*, 1987; Matthews, 1987).

The discovery by Hokin & Hokin (1955) that the turnover of the membrane phospholipid, phosphatidylinositol (PI), was stimulated by acetylcholine in the brain, was the first demonstration in the nervous system of the novel secondary messenger system known as the phosphatidylinositol system or PI system. This involves the receptor-mediated hydrolysis of membrane phosphatidylinositides to yield two secondary messengers: inositol triphosphate and diacylglycerol (Berridge, 1984). Since the initial studies by Hokin & Hokin, many neurotransmitter receptors have been identified as stimulating the PI system, and it is now considered one of the central regulatory mechanisms in neuronal tissue.

Receptor subtypes associated with the neurotransmitters acetylcholine and serotonin have been shown to activate either the PI or cAMP systems. Discussion of these neurotransmitters will therefore serve as illustrations of the initiation of these secondary messenger systems in the nervous system.

The neuropeptides are a group of putative neurotransmitters that have come under intense investigation in recent years. Two prominent neuropeptides identified within the central and peripheral nervous system are vasoactive intestinal peptide (VIP) and substance P. The secondary messenger responses associated with these two neuropeptides will be discussed in relation to their proposed modulatory role in the nervous system.

An interesting new development in the field of neurobiology is the finding that more than one putative neurotransmitter can be contained within the same neurone. In several instances one of these putative neurotransmitters is seen to have a modulatory effect on the other. Consideration of such interactions will be made in this chapter, together with the question of whether the mechanism can be described by changes in the secondary messenger responses.

6.2 Neurotransmitter sensitive secondary messenger systems

6.2.1 *Adenylate and guanylate cyclase*
A hormone- and neurotransmitter-sensitive adenylate cyclase system consists of three functional components: the receptor, the adenylate cyclase enzyme; and a transducer component termed a G-protein due to its guanine nucleotide-binding properties (Ross & Gilman, 1977; Ross *et al.*, 1978). Activation of the adenylate cyclase results in the formation of cAMP from ATP. Cyclic AMP is then degraded by a specific phosphodiesterase, thereby terminating the secondary messenger signal.

Receptor-binding of a neurotransmitter results in a conformational change in the receptor. The receptor is then able to associate with an inactive G-protein. In the inactive form, the guanine nucleotide binding site of the G-protein is occupied by GDP. On association with the neurotransmitter/receptor complex, the G-protein substitutes GDP for GTP and is subsequently activated. The G-protein dissociates from the neurotransmitter/receptor complex and binds to an adenylate cyclase enzyme, thereby activating the enzyme. The system is 'switched off' by hydrolysis of the GTP to GDP by an endogenous GTP'ase activity associated with the G-protein (Figure 6.1).

The above sequence of events describes the activation of adenylate by receptors that are positively linked to the enzyme. Receptors can however be negatively coupled, where receptor occupation results in the activation of an inhibitory G-protein termed Gi, with subsequent inhibition of cyclase activity.

Once synthesised, cAMP mediates numerous physiological reponses mainly via the activation of a cAMP-dependent protein kinase, an enzyme found in high concentrations in the brain (Nairn *et al.*, 1985).

Unlike adenylate cyclase, guanylate cyclase is a cytosolic enzyme, the stimulation of which results in the synthesis of cGMP from GTP. Degradation of cGMP is catalysed by a specific phosphodiesterase. As in the case of cAMP, many of the physiological responses of cGMP are mediated by activation of a cGMP-dependent protein kinase. The concentration of the protein kinase is generally low throughout the brain, with the exception of the cerebellum, an area where cGMP is thought to have modulatory functions (Nairn *et al.*, 1985)

Not all of the cellular effects of cGMP are mediated by protein phosphorylation. This is particularly true in the vertebrate photoreceptor, where cGMP has been shown to have a direct action on the ion channels involved in phototransduction (Matthews *et al.*, 1987).

6.2.2 *Phosphatidylinositide hydolysis*
In recent years the importance of the membrane phospholipids, phosphatidylinositides, in cellular function has become clear. These phospholipids make up a very small proportion of the total membrane phospholipid pool but their turnover, stimulated by a variety of neurotransmitters and hormones, has been shown to be instrumental in the control of cellular activity.

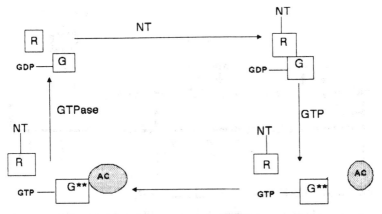

Fig. 6.1 Receptor-mediated activation of adenylate cyclase can be described in four steps: (1) receptor binding of the neurotransmitter or agonist results in the formation of a neurotransmitter/receptor/G-protein complex; (2) GDP is substituted for GTP at the guanine nucleotide binding site of the G-protein, resulting in the dissociation of the G-protein from the neurotransmitter/receptor/G-protein complex. The G-protein is now in its active form and is able (3) to associate with adenylate cyclase and thereby activating the enzyme; (4) the termination is the hydrolysis of GTP by an endogenous GTPase activity of the G-protein. NT, Neurotransmitter; R, receptor; G, inactive G-protein; G^{**}, activated G-protein; AC, adenylate cyclase.

Receptor-binding of a neurotransmitter results in the activation of a specific membrane bound phosphodiesterase, phospholipase C. This enzyme catalyses the hydrolysis of phosphatidylinositides to diacylglycerol and inositol triphosphate (Figure 6.2), both of which have been shown to act as secondary messengers in a number of cell types (for reviews see Berridge & Irvine, 1984; Berridge, 1984; Downes, 1986; Abdel-Latif, 1986; Osborne *et al.*, 1987). Diacylglycerol stimulates a Ca^{2+}/phospholipid-dependent protein kinase termed protein kinase C (Nishizuka, 1984). Substrates specific to protein kinase C include many neuronal components such as receptors (Huganir *et al.*, 1983) and neurotransmitter synthesising enzymes (Raese *et al.*, 1981). An important property of protein kinase C is that it can be stimulated by a group of compounds known as the tumour-promoting phorbol esters (Davis *et al.*, 1985) and by diacylglycerol analogues (Castagna *et al.*, 1982). This allows for the experimental stimulation

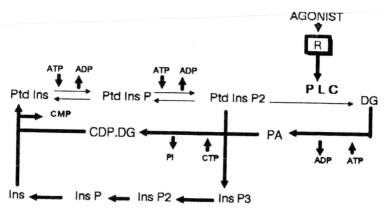

Fig. 6.2   Membrane phosphatidylinositol (Ptd Ins) is phosphorylated to phosphatidylinositol 4, phosphate (Ptd Ins P) and then to phosphatidylinositol 4,5, bisphosphate (Ptd Ins P2) by specific kinases in the membrane. On the binding of a neurotransmitter by the receptor, a membrane phosphodiesterase termed phospholipase C (PLC) is activated and hydrolyses Ptd Ins P2 to yield two secondary messengers; inositol triphosphate (Ins P3) and diacylglycerol (DG). Ins P3 is metabolised by dephosphorylation to inositol diphosphate (Ins P2), then inositol monophosphate (Ins P) and finally inositol (Ins). Inositol is then recycled back into the phosphatidylinositide pool. DG is phosphorylated to phosphatidic acid (PA) which is then primed by interaction with CTP to form cytidine diphosphate diacylglycerol (CDP.DG) and in this way recycled back into the phosphatidylinositide pool.

of just the diacylglycerol arm of this otherwise dual secondary messenger system. Deactivation of the protein kinase activity is effected by the phosphorylation of diacylglycerol by diacylglycerol kinase to phosphatidic acid which is then recycled into the membrane phosphatidylinositide pool (Figure 6.2).

Inositol triphosphate, the second component of this dual secondary messenger system, has been shown to mobilise intracellular calcium in a number of non-neuronal cell types (see Berridge & Irvine 1984; Abdel-Latif 1986). Whether the same action is seen in neuronal tissue is not clear and requires further investigation. The mechanism of deactivation of inositol triphosphate is its dephosphorylation to inositol, which is then recycled back into the phosphatidylinositide pool (Figure 6.2).

6.3 **Serotonin-stimulated secondary messenger systems**

Serotonin is a well-established neurotransmitter of the CNS. The majority of serotonergic cell bodies are concentrated in the raphe nuclei situated in the brain stem and their projections end in a diffuse distribution of nerve terminals throughout the CNS (Azmitia, 1978). Serotonin is seen mainly as a modulator of neuronal activity and has been implicated in the control of a variety of central functions including appetite, arousal, sleep, and pain perception (Bradley & Costa, 1984; Osborne, 1972). Furthermore dysfunction of serotonergic systems has been linked with clinical conditions such as depression and Alzheimers disease (Crow *et al.*, 1984).

6.3.1 *Stimulation of adenylate cyclase*

On the basis of the binding affinities of agonists and antagonists Peroutka & Snyder (1979) classified serotonergic receptors into two basic subtypes: 5HT-1 and 5HT-2. In this study the 5HT-1 subtype was shown to have a high affinity for serotonin and other agonists whilst the 5HT-2 receptor was shown to have a high affinity for antagonists (Peroutka & Synder, 1979).

The presence of a serotonin-sensitive adenylate cyclase in the brain was first detected in newborn rats (Von Hungen *et al.*, 1974). Initial investigations into the serotonin receptor subtype that might be linked to adenylate cyclase made use of the sensitivity such receptors would have to guanine nucleotides. Work carried out on non-neuronal tissue demonstrated that GTP decreased the binding affinities of receptors that were linked to adenylate cyclase. The locus of the GTP activity was shown to be the G-protein (Limbird, 1981). Application of GTP to adult rat brain homogenates decreases the binding of ^{3}H-5HT and also the potency of various agonists in the displacement of ^{3}H-5HT (Peroutka *et al.*, 1979; Mallat & Hamon, 1982). These studies indicated that the 5HT-1 receptor in the brain was linked to a G-protein and therefore was the receptor associated with the stimulation of adenylate cyclase. Further evidence came from direct studies on rat brain synaptosomes where nanomolar amounts of serotonin were demonstrated to stimulate adenylate cyclase activity (Fillion *et al.*, 1979a and b).

There is a good correlation between the distribution of serotonin-stimulated adenylate cyclase and serotonergic nerve terminals, which suggests that serotonin released *in vivo* does have an action on the serotonin-sensitive adenylate cyclase systems identified in homogenate and synaptosomal preparations. However the pre- or postsynaptic location of the receptors can not be established from these studies. One approach used to determine the pre- or postsynaptic location of a variety of central and peripheral receptors is that of specific neuronal destruction. By surgical lesions or neurotoxin action, removal of specific nerve terminals can be effected. The receptors lost by denervation must have been located on the terminals of the destroyed neurones, therefore indicating that these receptors are presynaptic. The remaining receptor population are either presynaptically located on the terminals of neurones not destroyed or postsynaptically located. In the case of 5HT-1 sites in the hippocampus, specific serotonergic lesions resulting from surgical intervention or application of the neurotoxin 5,7-dihydroxytryptamine resulted in an increase in the serotonin-sensitive adenylate cyclase activity (Barbaccia *et al.*, 1983). This is consistent with the postsynaptic location of serotonin receptors. The increase in adenylate cyclase sensitivity seen following serotonergic denervation is described as supersensitivity, which is observed in many postsynaptic receptor-mediated events following depletion of neurotransmitter levels.

However, the relationship between the serotonin receptor and adenylate cyclase has been complicated by binding studies that have revealed a number of 5HT-1 subtypes namely: 5HT-1a, 5HT-1b (Pedigo *et al.*, 1981) and 5HT-1c (Conn *et al.*, 1986). The 5HT-1a subtype is thought to be positively linked to adenylate cyclase, while 5HT-1b receptors may be negatively linked to adenylate cyclase in the rat brain (see Sanders-Bush, 1987) (Table 6.1).

6.3.2 *Stimulation of phosphatidylinositide hydrolysis*
As mentioned above, 5HT-2 receptors can be identified by their high affinity for antagonists such as spiperone, mianserin and ketanserin. Binding studies have demonstrated 5HT-2 sites in a number of brain areas but they are particularly concentrated in the frontal cortex (Leysen *et al.*, 1984). Central 5HT-2 receptors

Table 6.1   *Serotonin receptors and their secondary messengers*

Receptor	Secondary messenger	Location
5HT-1a	Positively coupled adenylate cyclase	Guinea-pig and rat hippocampus
5HT-1b	Negatively coupled to adenylate cyclase	Guinea-pig and rat hippocampus and cultured neurones
5HT-1c	Coupled to PI system	Rat and pig choroid plexus
5HT-2	Coupled to PI system	Rabbit retina and iris–ciliary body complex, rat cerebral cortex and platelets

show very similar characteristics to those in non-neuronal tissues, in particular blood platelets where binding of serotonin to 5HT-2 sites is thought to mediate serotonin-induced platelet activation. Platelets have thus provided a model for the study of 5HT-2 receptors and the secondary messenger systems associated with them.

Serotonin-mediated phosphatidylinositide hydrolysis has been identified in platelets (Schächter *et al.*, 1984) where this response is associated with an elevation of intracellular calcium and activation of protein kinase C (Affolter *et al.*, 1984; de Courcelles *et al.*, 1984). The selective 5HT-2 antagonist, ketanserin, was a potent inhibitor of the serotonin response, therefore indicating that the 5HT-2 receptor in rabbit platelets is linked to the PI system (Schächter *et al.*, 1984), and suggesting that the same might be true in the nervous system. Investigation of the cerebral cortex revealed a serotonin-stimulated turnover of phosphatidylinositides that was blocked by the potent 5HT-2 antagonists pizotifen and ketanserin (Conn & Sanders-Bush, 1984). Similarly in the retina (Cutcliffe & Osborne, 1987), and in the iris–ciliary body (Tobin *et al.*, 1988), 5HT-2 receptors linked to the PI system have been described (Figure 6.3). It appears therefore that the analogy between 5HT-2 receptors in platelets and the nervous tissue holds true with regard to the secondary messenger

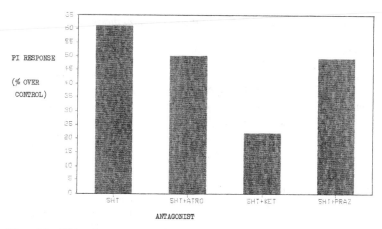

Fig. 6.3 This shows serotonin-stimulated PI response in the rabbit iris–ciliary body complex. Receptor characterisation was performed by blocking the response with various antagonists. The potent 5HT-2 receptor antagonist ketanserin (KET), $10-6\,mol\,L^{-1}$, reduced the response significantly whereas the alpha$_1$-adrenergic antagonist prazosin (PRAZ), $10-6\,mol\,L^{-1}$, and the muscarinic antagonist atropine (ATRO), $10-6\,mol\,L^{-1}$, had very little effect on the serotonin response. This indicates that the serotonin stimulated PI response maybe mediated via 5HT-2 receptors.

system utilised (Table 6.1) However, whether diacylglycerol activates protein kinase C or inositol triphosphate mobilises intracellular calcium in nervous tissue, as they do in platelets, is yet to be to established. Kandell & Nahorski (1984) have, however, demonstrated that the serotonin PI response in the cerebral cortex is dependent on the levels of intracellular calcium. Berridge & Irvine (1984) proposed that if the action of a secondary messenger is to be a regulator of intracellular calcium levels then its generation most be independent of calcium concentrations. The demonstration of a calcium dependency for the generation of inositol phosphates stimulated by serotonin, in the cerebral cortex, suggests that in this instance inositol triphosphate may not be involved in the mobilisation of intracellular calcium.

6.4 Acetylcholine stimulated secondary messenger systems

The acetylcholine receptor has been classified into two main receptor subtypes; nicotinic and muscarinic, because of their relative affinities for the agonists nicotine and muscarine respectively. The cholinergic-nicotinic receptor has been isolated from a variety of tissues, including the electric organ of *Torpedo*, and the neuromuscular junction, and has been found to be an ion channel. Binding of acetylcholine to the nicotinic receptor results in the opening of the ion channel and therefore an increase in membrane permeability to sodium and potassium (Changeux *et al.*, 1984; Mishina, 1985).

The muscarinic receptor itself may be classified into four subtypes on the basis of its different stimulatory effects on secondary messenger systems and ion permeabilities (Table 6.2). Muscarinic receptors located on hippocampal pyramidal cells and postganglionic sympathetic neurones are linked to potassium ion channels known as M channels. In the cerebellum, muscarinic receptors are linked to guanylate cyclase, where they stimulate the synthesis of cGMP. In various brain regions and in neuronal cultures, muscarinic receptors have been shown to be negatively linked to adenylate cyclase via a Gi-protein. Therefore the occupation of the receptor will result in decreased cAMP synthesis. Finally there is evidence demonstrating muscarinic receptor-mediated hydrolysis of phosphatidylinositol in a number of brain areas (see Levine *et al.*, 1985).

We will focus attention on the muscarinic-mediated inhibition of adenylate cyclase and the stimulation of the PI system.

6.4.1 *Muscarinic inhibition of adenylate cyclase*
Opiate, alpha$_2$-adrenergic and cholinergic muscarinic receptors are among those receptors that are negatively linked to adenylate cyclase in the nervous system. They all share very similar properties and are therefore thought to inhibit cyclase activity through the same mechanism (Klee *et al.*, 1984). Muscarinic inhibition of adenylate cyclase has been identified in striatal synaptic membrane preparations and in the neuronal cell culture NG108–15 (Olianas *et al.*, 1983; Hughes *et al.*, 1984). Neuronal cell cultures have been used extensively in the study of the mechanism of

Table 6.2   *Acetylcholine receptors and their secondary messengers*

Receptor	Secondary messenger	Location
Nicotinic	Ion gate	Neuromuscular junction and electric organ of *Torpedo*
Muscarinic	Linked to K^+	Hippocampus and cultured neurones
	Negatively linked to adenylate cyclase	Striatum and cultured neurones
	Linked to guanylate cyclase	Cerebellum
	Linked to PI system	Rat and guinea-pig brain

muscarinic action, and have provided strong evidence for the presence of a Gi-protein (Hughes *et al.*, 1984).

The G-proteins are considered to be trimers of heterogeneous subunits, α,β,γ, where the β- and γ-subunits of the Gs and Gi-proteins are identical but the α-subunits are heterogenous and termed αs and αi respectively. The α-subunit is the location of the GTP/GDP binding site and the GTPase activity involved in the deactivation process. Activation of the G-protein by association with a neurotransmitter/receptor complex consists of two distinct events; the substitution of GDP for GTP at the α-subunit and the dissociation of the trimer to an α-subunit and a β,γ-complex. The α-subunit then binds with adenylate cyclase either activating (αs) or inhibiting (αi) cyclase activity.

The β-, γ-subunits resulting from the activation of the Gi-protein can also inhibit cyclase activity by the binding of free αs-subunits to form a $\alpha s\beta\gamma$-complex and in this way preventing the association of the αs-unit with adenylate cyclase (Codina *et al.*, 1984). This 'mopping up' of the αs-subunit is thought to be the primary mechanism of action of inhibitory neurotransmitters.

The important feature to recognise in this mechanism is that muscarinic receptors may be able to inhibit adenylate cyclase activities that have been stimulated by other neurotransmitters. This suggests a modulatory role for muscarinic receptors on the levels of cAMP elevated by neurotransmitters that are positively linked to adenylate cyclase. An example of this modulatory function is seen in the striatum. Synaptosomal preparations from the rat striatum contain a dopamine-sensitive adenylate cyclase which is stimulated upon occupation of DA-1 dopamine receptors. Acetylcholine reduced both the basal and the dopamine stimulated cAMP levels, indicating that the adenylate cyclase sensitive to dopamine and acetylcholine is located on the same postsynaptic membrane and that they are functionally coupled (Olianas *et al.*, 1983).

6.4.2 *Muscarinic stimulation of the PI system*
Acetylcholine was first demonstrated to increase the turnover of phosphatidylinositides in the guinea-pig brain by Hokin & Hokin (1955). It is now known to stimulate the PI system in a variety of areas including the striatum, cerebral cortex, hippocampus and iris–ciliary body complex, where the responses are blocked by the potent muscarinic antagonist atropine.

The muscarinic receptor is thought to have two affinity states, a high and a low affinity state. By comparing the concentrations of agonists required to stimulate the PI response to half its maximal stimulation (EC_{50}) with the binding constant (K) for that agonist to the high and low affinity states, it was possible to identify which of the affinity states was associated with the PI response. Using this approach it was found that agonists such as oxotremorine and acetylcholine stimulated the PI response by occupation of the low affinity state receptor (Fisher, 1986).

There is considerable variation between the potencies of agonists seen in different regions of the CNS. Full agonists, oxotremorine and carbamylcholine, were more potent stimulators of the PI system in the neostriatum than in the cerebral cortex. Also the partial agonist bethanechol displayed a potency in the neostriatum four times that in the hippocampus or cerebral cortex (Fisher & Bartus, 1985). This suggested that different muscarinic receptor subtypes are linked to the PI system and that these receptor subtypes had a specific distribution in the CNS, thus explaining the disparity between the agonists potencies observed in various brain regions (Fisher & Bartus, 1985).

The question of muscarinic receptor subtypes is further complicated by binding studies that have identified two receptor subtypes, M1 and M2, from the binding of the antagonist pirenzapine (Hammer & Giachetti, 1982). Attempts to ascribe secondary messenger responses to the activation of M1 or M2 subtypes have been unsuccessful due to the contradictary results obtained from different tissues. For example, pirenzapine inhibited the PI response in the guinea-pig cerebral cortex and hippocampus suggesting that the muscarinic PI response was mediated by M1 receptors (Fisher & Bartus, 1985), whereas in the neostriatum and in non-neuronal tissue, such as the parotid gland, pirenzapine had a low potency for the inhibition of the PI response (Gil & Wolfe, 1984; Fisher & Bartus, 1985). These results illustrate the importance of being able to associate a cellular or physiological response to a receptor subtype that has been identified by ligand-binding studies. Until such an association is demonstrated, the receptor subtypes identified from binding studies must be considered as putative subtypes, as they may be artifacts of the binding preparation with no physiological significance.

Although muscarinic receptor stimulation of the PI system has been demonstrated in the brain, it is still not clear whether this results in the activation of protein kinase C and calcium mobilisation, as suggested by the work on non-neuronal tissue. Initial experiments with a neuroblastoma cell line MCNB-1 preloaded with a fluorescent calcium indicator Quin-2 have demonstrated that on application of muscarinic agonists there is an increase in intracellular calcium (Fisher, 1986). A direct association between the elevated calcium levels and PI hydrolysis has, however, not been established.

6.5 Neuropeptide-stimulated secondary messenger systems

Peptides such as cholecystokinin (pancreozymin), vasoactive intestinal peptide (VIP), bombesin and substance P were isolated in the gastrointestinal tract before their localisation in neuronal tissue. With the characterisation of substance P from the bovine hypothalamic tissue (Chang & Leeman, 1970) the concept of dual occurrence of peptides in the gut and brain was born. However not all neuropeptides are gut–brain peptides. The enkephalins, for example, have no endocrinological function in the gut but are considered to be neuropeptides in a number of peripheral and central sites.

Preceding many of the advances in neuroscience are improvements or new developments in experimental techniques. In the case of the neuropeptides the technological advance was in the form of immunocytochemistry and radioimmunoassay (RIA). The size of most of the neuropeptides is such as to make them potent immunogens. Antisera raised against the peptides can then be used for immunocytochemical or radioimmunoassay mapping of peptide distribution in the brain. These studies revealed not only the diversity of neuropeptides but also their wide distribution in the CNS.

Due to their slow time course of action, the relatively large distance between the size of release and target sites, and the lack of a specific rapid degradative pathway the neuropeptides are generally not thought to be neurotransmitters but demonstrate characteristics associated with neuromodulators (see Krieger, 1983). What is meant by the term neuromodulator has been discussed elsewhere (Osborne, 1980). The sites at which a neuromodulator might act are numerous and include the synthesis, storage and release of a neurotransmitter and the postsynaptic response of a neurotransmitter.

Two particularly well characterised neuropeptides are substance P and VIP and it these two that will be briefly considered.

6.5.1 *Substance P*

Substance P is thought to be a primary neurotransmitter candidate for sensory neurones. At the central site, terminals from the sensory ganglion neurones project into laminae II and III of the dorsal horn of the spinal cord (substantia gelatinosa), which are areas associated with pain and temperature perception. At this site, substance P is thought to be the neurotransmitter associated with pain perception. The peripheral functions of this peptide have been investigated in the rabbit iris, where it causes contraction of the sphincter smooth muscle and closure of the pupil {miosis} (Bito *et al.*, 1982) in response to noxious stimulation. The mechanism underlying this response is thought to be the receptor activation of the PI system, since substance P-mediated hydrolysis of phosphatidylinositides is associated with a strong contractile response in the rabbit iris sphincter smooth muscle (Yousufzai *et al.*, 1986). It is suggested that substance P within the sensory neurones innervating the iris is released on the application of a noxious stimulant resulting the production of inositol triphosphate. Subsequent mobilisation of intracellular calcium initiates smooth muscle contraction (Yousufzai *et al.*, 1986).

Further evidence for substance P receptors linked to the PI system has come from studies in the guinea-pig intestine where substance P was shown to increase the levels of inositol triphosphate and cause smooth muscle contraction (Watson, 1984; Holzer & Lippe, 1985). In this preparation substance P had no effect on the cAMP levels (Watson, 1984).

6.5.2 *Vasoactive intestinal peptide*

The first indication that VIP receptors in the brain were linked to adenylate cyclase came from the studies by Deschodt-Lanckman *et al.* (1977) on guinea-pig brain synaptosomal preparations. VIP receptors coupled to adenylate cyclase have since been demonstrated in a number of central (Quik *et al.*, 1978; Borghi *et al.*, 1979) and peripheral sites (Mittag & Tormay, 1985), where VIP is considered to have a neuromodulatory role.

Recent studies have identified a new type of VIP receptor linked to the PI system. Accumulation of inositol phosphates was observed in the rat superior cervical ganglion following incubation with VIP (Audigier *et al.*, 1986). Binding studies using ^{125}I-VIP have demonstrated a two state receptor model where there is a time-dependent transition between high and low affinity VIP binding states (Staun-Olsen *et al.*, 1982). Audigier *et al.* (1986) suggest that the dominant receptor in the superior cervical ganglion is the low affinity state receptor and that in this state the receptor is linked to the PI system.

6.6 **Cotransmission**

The original concept of neurotransmission as developed by Langley, Dales, Elliot and Loewi presumed that a neurone utilises the same neurotransmitter at all of its synapses. This concept was formally outlined by Eccles in the mid 1950s: he described it as

'Dale's principle'. However, by the use of immunological and autoradiographical techniques there are now many examples where more than one putative neurotransmitter has been localised within the same neurone (see Osborne, 1982a); a situation termed coexistence. These studies have in recent years brought the validity of Dale's principle into doubt (see Cuello, 1982).

Demonstration of coexistence is in itself not sufficent evidence for cotransmission. Cotransmission requires that both putative neurotransmitters are synthesised, stored and released from the same neurone and that they have a postsynaptic action. Adenosine triphosphate (ATP) and noradrenaline, released simultaneously from sympathetic postganglionic fibres innervating the guinea-pig vas deferens, have been shown to act as neurotransmitters at the smooth musculature (Westfall *et al.*, 1978). This is one of the few instances where both neuroactive agents fulfil the criteria of neurotransmitters and it is, therefore, a clear example of cotransmission in the peripheral nervous system.

The complexity of the vertebrate CNS has hampered investigations of cotransmission at central sites. Consequently, the only convincing evidence for cotransmission in the CNS has come from studies on the snail brain. Each cerebral ganglion of the snail *Helix* contains a large serotonergic cell termed the giant serotonin cell (GSC). The cell forms monosynaptic connections with follower cells in the buccal ganglion. It has been proposed that acetylcholine is present in the GSC and electrophysiological studies indicate that acetylcholine is coreleased with serotonin resulting in a change in membrane conductance at the buccal follower cells (see Osborne, 1982b).

The coexistence of classical neurotransmitters with neuropeptides is of particular interest as one might predict that the neuropeptide acts as a modulator of the neurotranmitters action. Electron microscopical studies have demonstrated that in the majority of cases the neuropeptides are stored in large dense core vesicles, while neurotransmitters are stored in smaller clear vesicles. This allows for the possibility of differential release of the coexisting agents, determined by physiological conditions such as the rate of nerve firing.

One of the first examples of neuropeptide–neurotransmitter coexistence was the presence of substance P in serotonergic cell bodies of the raphe nuclei (Chan–Palay, 1982). Projections from these neurones were shown to terminate in the ventral horn of the spinal cord (Gilbert *et al.*, 1982), where serotonin and substance P are stored in the same large dense core vesicles (Pelletier *et al.*, 1981). Costorage of the two neuroactive agents indicates simultaneous release on nerve stimulation. Substance P has been shown to increase the number and decrease the affinity of serotonergic binding sites in the ventral horn (Agnati *et al.*, 1983), suggesting that it may act as a modulator of serotonergic transmission. However, there is no evidence demonstrating the release of substance P and serotonin, nor a postsynaptic effect.

Combined immunocytochemistry and histochemistry have demonstrated the presence of VIP in the parasympathetic neurones innervating the cat submandibular gland (Lundberg *et al.*, 1979). There is a close association between these nerve fibres and the acinar cells and blood vessels. Acetylcholine acts as a neurotransmitter at the acinar cells and blood vessels stimulating salivary secretion and vasodilation, via the activation of muscarinic receptors (Lundberg, 1981).

Electron microscopy studies have revealed that VIP is stored within large dense core vesicles and acetylcholine in small clear vesicles. Low frequency (2 Hz) stimulation of the parasympathetic nerves results in the release of acetylcholine, and at high frequencies (10 Hz) there is a simultaneous release of acetylcholine and VIP, demonstrating that there can be differential release of coexisting neuroactive agents. VIP has a modulatory function at the acinar cells, potentiating the acetylcholine effect, and a transmitter function at the vasculature, causing vasodilation (Lundberg, 1981; Lundberg & Hökfelt, 1983). VIP is thought to potentiate acetylcholines effects at the acinar cell by inducing a shift from the low to the high affinity states, thereby increasing the affinity of acetylcholine receptors (Lundberg, 1982).

6.6.1 *Molecular mechanism for cotransmission*
As can be seen from Figure 6.4, secondary messenger pathways generated by two different neurotransmitters can interact at a number of levels. As mentioned above, putative neurotransmitters can alter the density and affinities of receptor populations. The mechanism of such action might be the activation of protein

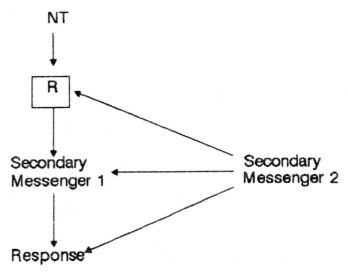

Fig. 6.4 The various points at which a secondary messenger generated by one neurotransmitter can interact with a secondary messenger response generated by another neurotransmitter is illustrated. Secondary messenger 2 might interact at the level of the receptor (R), the metabolism of secondary messenger 1 or the physiological response of secondary messenger 1 {see text}.

kinase phosphorylation of specific sites on the receptor. Alternatively, the secondary messenger could potentiate or attenuate the sythesis of other secondary messengers. This may be due to activation of a regulatory protein or by direct interaction with the synthesising enzymes. An example of the latter is the $Ca^{2+}/$ calmodulin activation of adenylate cyclase in the brain (Brostorm *et al.*, 1979). Thirdly, secondary messengers have been shown to increase the activity of enzymes involved in the metabolism of other secondary messengers, for example cGMP may regulate cAMP levels by stimulating the activity of specific cAMP/ phosphodiesterase (see Lincoln & Corbin, 1983). Finally, secondary messenger pathways can interact at the level of the physiological response. For example, a phosphoprotein might be phosphorylated by two protein kinases each activated by different secondary messenger pathways. This might represent a convergence of the two pathways, if each of the protein kinases phosphorylates the same site on the protein, or a point of modulation, if each phosphorylates a different site on the protein. Many of the substrate proteins for cAMP-dependent protein kinase are phosphorylated at the same sites by cGMP-dependent protein kinase (Nestler & Greengard, 1984), although in most cases the physiological significance is unknown.

It is plausible that coexisting putative neurotransmitters, simultaneously released onto the postsynaptic membrane, interact at one of the levels discussed above. This hypothesis is particularly attractive if one of the coexisting neuroactive agents is suspected of having a neuromodulatory role – and therefore of potentiating or attenuating the postsynaptic action of the primary neurotransmitter.

6.7 Concluding remarks

Although neuroscientists are aware of the complexities of neuronal communication, our knowledge is not yet at a stage where we can fully understand this fundamental process. The generation of secondary messengers is of undisputed importance in neuronal communication but in the majority of cases the physiological consequence of changes in intracellular levels of secondary messengers is unknown. It is therefore clear that a great deal of experimentation is still needed to resolve the question of how neurones communicate.

Acknowledgement

We thank the Wellcome Trust for their financial support.

6.8 Further reading

(Other literature is listed in the compiled references at the end of the book.)

Abdel-Latif, A. A. (1986). Calcium-mobilising receptors, polyphosphoinositides and the generation of secondary messengers. *Physiological Reviews*, **38**, 227–72.

Limbird, L. L. (1981). Activation and attenuation of adenylate cyclase. *Biochemical Journal*, **195**, 1–13.

Lundberg, J. M. & Hokflet, T. (1983). Coexistence of peptides & classical neurotransmitters. *Trends in Neurosciences*, **6**, 325–33.

Nestler, E. J. & Greengard, P. (1984). *Protein phosphorylation in the nervous system*. John Wiley, New York.

Nishizuka, Y. (1984). The role of protein kinase C in cell surface signal transduction and tumour promotion. *Nature*, **308**, 693–8.

Osborne, N. N. (1982). *Dales principle and communication between neurones*. Pergamon Press, Oxford.

Receptors on glia: their role in neuronal function

H. Ghazi and N. N. Osborne   Nuffield Laboratory of Ophthalmology, Oxford

7.1 Introduction

Generally, neurones are in direct functional contact with other neurones only at synapses. The remainder of the nerve cell is surrounded by and separated from glial cells by extracellular spaces that appear 10–12 nm wide in electron microscopy. As early as 1928, it was evident to Cajal, from anatomical evidence, that this close association forms the basis of a symbiotic relationship between neurones and glial cells in the nervous system. This concept was pursued by Hydén (1967) as he and his colleagues described, in a series of (perhaps controversial) studies, reciprocal changes which take place between certain neurones and their surrounding glia during various functional states. They provided indirect evidence suggesting that glial cells support neurones by a transfer of nutrients and macromolecules such as RNA (Hydén, 1962; Hydén & Lange, 1962).

In recent years, it has become evident that a neurone–glia relationship (see Table 7.1) begins during development of the nervous system and persists throughout life, as seen, for example, in the directional guidance of the 'radial glia cells' for the young neurones, malfunction of glial cell metabolism leading to failure of effective neurotransmission, and glial cell proliferation in response to cerebral injury. This, however, is not unexpected, since studies have shown that astrocytes, on their own, constitute a large portion of the volume of the mammalian brain cortex (Pope, 1978) and their relative number, compared to neurones, is especially high in adult mammals (Bass *et al.*, 1971).

Table 7.1   *Neurone – glia relationship*

Neurones are surrounded by glial cells (EC space $\simeq$ 10–12 nm)
Directional guidance of the 'radial glial cells' for the young neurones
Potassium buffering in the extracellular space
Active uptake of various neuroactive substances by glial cells
Ng-CAM, N-CAM and NGF, etc.
Glial proliferation in response to cerebral injury
Malfunction of glial cells leading to failure of effective transmission
Receptors on glial cells
Neuronal-induced glycogenolysis in glial cells

Furthermore, in addition to removing potassium from the extracellular fluid, it has been observed that glial cells, both *in vitro* and *in vivo*, actively take up, synthesise, metabolise and/or release some of the neuroactive substances suspected of having a role in synaptic transmission. These putative transmitters include glutamate, aspartate, GABA, taurine, hypotaurine, glycine, noradrenaline, dopamine and serotonin (see Hansson, 1986). These glial properties, which may obviously modify the neuronal microenvironment, represent one facet of neurone–glia interactions. Another feature of the relationship is suggested by reports demonstrating the presence of various putative transmitter receptors on glial cells (see Table 7.2). Indeed, muscarinic cholinergic (Repke & Maderspach, 1982; Cambray-Deakin *et al.*, 1985), adrenergic (Van Calken *et al.*, 1978; McCarthy & de Vellis, 1979; Hosli & Hosli, 1982; Hosli *et al.*, 1982; Hirata *et al.*, 1983), dopaminergic (Henn *et al.*, 1977; Hansson *et al.*, 1984), histaminergic (Hosli & Hosli, 1984; Hosli *et al.*, 1984) and serotonergic (Hertz *et al.*, 1979; Fillion *et al.*, 1980, 1983; Cambray-Deakin *et al.*, 1985) putative receptors have been demonstrated in intact or cultured glial cells.

Neurones may thus be able to communicate and interact with as well as to influence glial cells receptors. The present chapter will attempt to describe the biochemical events which have been reported as occurring subsequent to activation of these glial receptors in relation to the general functioning of the nervous system.

Table 7.2 *Substances which increase the accumulation of inositol phosphates in glia*

	Putative receptor
Carbachol	Muscarinic
Noradrenaline	Alpha
Serotonin	$5\text{-}HT_2$
Histamine	??

7.2 Glial cells and second messengers

In Chapter 6, the mechanisms by which second messengers, namely cAMP, inositol triphosphate and diacylglycerol, are produced within the cell have been described. Using primary non-neuronal (Muller cells) rabbit retinal cultures we have identified muscarinic cholinergic and α-adrenergic receptors linked to inositol phosphate metabolism. Carbachol and noradrenaline stimulated the accumulation of inositol phosphates in these cells in a dose-dependent manner. These responses were pharmacologically characterised and shown to be mediated by muscarinic-cholinergic and α_1-adrenergic receptors, respectively (Ghazi & Osborne, 1988). In a similar study, Pearce *et al.* (1985a) have reported increased accumulation of inositol phosphates in astrocyte-enriched cultures prepared from newborn rat cortex, following the addition of carbachol, noradrenaline and serotonin to these cultures. As in the study with retinal cultures, the carbachol- and noradrenaline-mediated responses were found to be elicited via muscarinic cholinergic and α_1-adrenergic receptors; the serotonin response was not characterised (Pearce *et al.*, 1985a). In human astrocytoma cells, stimulation of muscarinic receptors also evoked an increase in the accumulation of inositol phosphates (Masters *et al.*, 1984). These studies clearly indicate the presence of a number of different types of functional transmitter receptors on glial cells (see Table 7.3 and Figure 7.1), which are linked to the phosphatidylinositol second messenger system. At present, there is little evidence concerning the functional significance of the increased production of inositol phosphates in glial cells. The activation of lipid phosphates by various transmitters has been shown, however, to increase intracellular

Table 7.3 *Substances increasing the accumulation of cAMP in glial cells*

	Putative Receptor
Noradrenaline	β
Serotonin	5-HT$_1$
Dopamine	DA'1'
Adenosine	A'1'
VIP	??
Glucagon	??
PGE$_1$	??

Ca^{2+} concentration by releasing it from ATP-dependent, non-mitochondrial pools (Streb *et al.*, 1983) as well as activating various Ca^{2+}, Ca^{2+}/calmodulin and protein kinase C (PKC)-dependent proteins within the cell (Berridge, 1984; England, 1986). Thus, it appears as if extracellular signals (or first messengers) can alter protein phosphorylation in glial cells by activating the receptors linked to the inositol phosphate system. This might lead to the modulation of glial membrane conductance, active transport, signal–receptor interaction and other glial functions by phosphorylating the appropriate proteins. Two speculative examples highlighting some of the possible functional aspect of this system in glial cells in relation to neurones will now be discussed.

It is generally accepted that intracellular glycogen breakdown is initiated by the production of cAMP within the cell (see next section). However a recent investigation by Pearce *et al.* (1985b) has demonstrated that stimulation of alpha-adrenergic receptors increases glycogenolysis in astrocyte-enriched cultures. One might speculate that the increased accumulation of inositol phosphates induced by the activation of α_1-adrenergic receptors in glial cells, may be partly responsible for the induction of glycogenolysis within glial cells. Another example occurs in the chicken brain glial cultures, where Kasa *et al.* (1984) have demonstrated that activation of the muscarinic cholinergic receptors in these cultures leads to the release of choline from these glial cells. It is thus conceivable that the activation of these muscarinic receptors by cholinergic agonists increases the accumulation of inositol phosphates, which would subsequently trigger the release

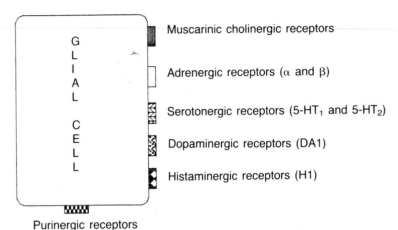

Fig. 7.1   The various transmitter receptors which have been established on glial cells using electrophysiological, binding and biochemical techniques.

of choline. Obviously, this would increase the availability of choline in the extracellular medium, thus considerably influencing the synthesis of acetylcholine in neuronal cells located in the vicinity.

It has been well established in the nervous system that a number of putative transmitters elicit their effects upon neurones via a cAMP-mediated mechanism (Gilman, 1972; Van Calker & Hamprecht, 1980). A multitude of evidence now exists, which indicates that some of these active substances elicit a similar increase in cyclic nucleotides in glial cells (see Kimelberg, 1988). Noradrenaline and isoproterenol increased the intracellular concentration of cAMP 100-fold or more in fetal rat brain glial cultures, transformed astrocytes and clonal lines of glial tumour cells. These responses were blocked by β-adrenergic receptor blockers, while phentolamine, an α-adrenergic antagonist, was ineffective (Clark & Perkins, 1971; Gilman & Nirenberg, 1971; Gilman & Schrier, 1972; Browning *et al.*, 1974; Cummins *et al.*, 1983). Although α-adrenergic receptor agonists did not affect basal levels of cAMP in primary cultures of glia, they modulated the β-adrenergic induced response which involves cAMP. Concurrent activation of these cultures with phenylephrine, an α-adrenergic receptor agonist, decreased the cAMP response to noradrenaline, adenosine and prostaglandin E_1. This modulatory effect of α-adrenergic agents was found not to be caused by activating the cAMP-dependent phosphodiesterase (McCarthy & de Vellis, 1978). Dopamine was also shown to increase cAMP levels in several lines of glia, however this response was blocked more substantially by propranolol (but not by phentolamine) than by neuroleptic drugs and therefore appeared to be modulated through β-adrenergic receptors. (Clark *et al.* 1975; Schubert *et al.*, 1976; Van Calker *et al.*, 1979). However, more recently, Hansson *et al.* (1984) have provided evidence for the existence of a genuine dopamine-stimulated cAMP formation in cerebral hemisphere primary cultures. This dopamine effect, which was dose- and time-dependent, was mimicked, to some extent, by the partial agonist apomorphine and was antagonized by fluphenazine. Moreover, the dopamine-induced stimulation was incompletely blocked by propranolol, suggesting a lesser interaction with β-adrenergic receptors than in previous studies. Interestingly, dopamine increased cAMP levels in astroglial cultures from the striatum, while no response was found in cultures arising from the brainstem, possibly suggesting some heterogeneity among astroglial cells. Although serotonin had no effect on adenylate cyclase activity in homogenates of rat glial tumour line (Jard *et al.*, 1972), recent studies have clearly demonstrated a class of serotonergic receptors in glial cell membrane fractions. The stimulation of these receptors with serotonin increases adenylate cyclase activity and is apparently serotonin-specific and clearly distinct from a dopamine-induced stimulation which was present in the same preparation. These receptors were also capable of binding [3H] serotonin with high affinity (Fillion *et al.*, 1980, 1983). Other substances which have been shown to stimulate cAMP formation in fetal rat brain cell cultures and in various glial cell lines include prostaglandin E_1, adenosine and histamine (Clark & Perkins, 1971; Gilman & Nirenberg, 1971; Gilman & Schrier, 1972).

Preliminary studies from our laboratory indicate that intracellular cAMP concentration in primary non-neuronal (Muller cells) rabbit retinal cultures is augmented, in a dose-dependent manner, by the exposure of these cultures to noradrenaline,

isoproterenol, serotonin and VIP, whereas carbachol, via muscarinic cholinergic receptors, attenuated the production of
cAMP within these cells. The noradrenaline and isoproterenol responses were found to be mediated by β-adrenergic receptors, as
only propranolol was capable of blocking these responses. The
serotonin-mediated response seems to be elicited via $5\text{-}HT_1$
receptors, since cholinergic, adrenergic, dopaminergic, histaminergic and $5\text{-}HT_2$ receptor antagonists were unable to block
the response, and 8-OH-DPAT induces a stimulatory response.
In relation to our study, a previous investigation using cultured
glial (Muller) cells of the chick retina, has demonstrated the
effects of two neuropeptides, VIP and glucagon upon these cells.
VIP, and to a lesser extent glucagon, stimulated the accumulation
of cAMP intracellularly in these cultures (Koh *et al.*, 1984). In
accordance with studies in our laboratory, the study by Koh *et al.*
(1984) found a stimulatory effect of isoproterenol on cAMP accumulation in cultured glial (Muller) cells. However, in contrast to
our results, they were unable to find such an effect by serotonin.

It has been established that the activation of adenylate cyclase
leads to increased production of cAMP within the cell, which has
been shown to activate one type of cAMP-dependent protein
kinase in the brain (Nestler & Greengard, 1984). This kinase is
responsible for the phosphorylation of various neuronal proteins.
Similarly to the activation of the phosphatidylinositol system,
activation of the adenylate cyclase enzyme by membrane receptors in glial cells is undoubtedly an important mechanism by
which neurones can communicate with glial cells. This has been
fairly well demonstrated in the case of the neuronal-induced
glycogen turnover in glial cells, which will be discussed in the
next section. Another example was supplied by Schwartz & Costa
(1977), where they have shown that the C6 glioma cell line
contains nerve growth factor (NGF) which can be released into
the extracellular medium. They reported that treatment of these
cells with β-adrenergic receptor agonists, such as isoproterenol,
noradrenaline and adrenaline, resulted in an intra- and extracellular increase in the content of NGF within 3 hours, whereas
α-adrenergic receptor agonists were ineffective. The response
was blocked by β- but not α-adrenergic receptor antagonists.
This increase in NGF was paralleled by a similar, although much

quicker, increase in intracellular cAMP concentration. Since the C6 glioma cell line contains a cAMP-dependent protein kinase (Opler & Makman, 1972), which is activated following stimulation of β-adrenergic receptors and this protein kinase is the only receptor protein for cAMP in brain, it was suggested that protein phosphorylation mediates the increase in NGF (Schwartz & Costa, 1977). It was also proposed that this activation of protein kinase could increase NGF content through a modulation of gene expression at the level of RNA translation, perhaps through nuclear translocation as has been suggested for the induction of tyrosine hydroxylase (Costa *et al.*, 1976). Functionally, these results may suggest that glial cells located adjacent to noradrenergic nerve terminals may be activated via their receptors during protracted increase of adrenergic neuronal activity, to produce and secrete NGF in the extracellular space (see Figure 7.2). The NGF can then either stimulate specific membrane receptors (Banerjee *et al.*, 1973; Frazier *et al.*, 1974) or can be taken up and transported to the soma by retrograde axonal transport (Hendry *et al.*, 1974; Stoeckel *et al.*, 1975), where it can induce the production of vital materials (Andres *et al.*, 1977).

7.3 Glial cells and glycogenolysis:

A prominent metabolic characteristic of glial cells relative to neurones is their higher rate of oxidative phosphorylation (Rapava *et al.*, 1973) and the higher activity of ATPase (Hamberger *et al.*, 1970; Sellinger *et al.*, 1971; Nagata *et al.*, 1974). Therefore, the glial cells demonstrate a greater capacity to accumulate and release energy in the form of ATP than do neurones. However, the neuronal energy requirements must be rather high, in order to maintain nerve impulses, ionic transport, the transport of macromolecules from the nucleus to the cytoplasm, and axonal flow. The glial cells having a smaller mass of cytoplasm and slow potentials, should have a considerably lower energy requirement. This, in addition to the fact that long astrocytic processes which contain fat and glycogen invaginate the neuronal soma, provided the basis of the earlier suggestions that the glial cells play a role in the supply of energy to neurones. This was supported by Hamberger & Hyden (1963), where excitation of

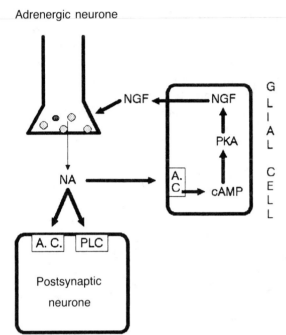

Fig. 7.2 Noradrenaline (NA) released from an adrenergic neurone may interact with receptors, on both glial cells and neurones, which may be linked to adenylate cyclase (A.C.) or phospholipase C (PLC). The stimulation of cAMP production in glial cells may lead to an activation of cAMP-dependent protein kinase (PKA) which in turn leads to the production and release of nerve growth factor (NGF).

the nervous system was accompanied by the activation of respiration and the inhibition of glycolysis (the Pasteur effect), in neurones, while the opposite simultaneously occurs (the Crabtree effect), in glial cells. Moreover, it was shown that neurones and their processes use mainly glucose as a substrate for metabolism, while a wide range of substrates, such as fatty and amino acids, can be utilised by glial cells (Balazs *et al.*, 1973). This seems to provide glial cells with a substantial advantage under conditions where carbohydrates are exhausted such as in hypoxia and increased functioning.

Various studies have, since then, reported that cAMP production, mediated by various agents, induces glycogen breakdown in primary astrocyte and astrocytoma cell cultures (Opler & Makman, 1972; Passonneau & Crites, 1976; Cummins *et al.*, 1983). Noradrenaline, adrenaline, histamine, dibutyryl cAMP and papaverine induced the degradation of glycogen in rat astrocytoma cells. These substances, except for histamine, stimulated adenylate cyclase and their glycogenolytic and enzymatic effects were blocked by propranolol. This suggests that cAMP mediates hormonally-induced glycogenolysis and that histamine acts in a manner different from noradrenaline and adrenaline. Similarly, Cummins *et al.* (1983) demonstrated that adrenergic agonists such as noradrenaline and isoproterenol caused an immediate and dose-dependent increase in intracellular cAMP levels in cultured astrocytes. Concurrently, with the initial phase of cAMP increase, conversion of phosphorylase b to a and glycogenolysis was observed. The increase in cAMP levels, phosphorylase conversion and glycogenolysis were simultaneously blocked by β-adrenergic blockers, but not α-adrenergic blocking agents (see Figure 7.3). Other studies have indicated that addition of noradrenaline to cultured glioblastoma cells results in an inhibition of uptake of radioactive glucose from the medium. In addition, if these cells are previously labelled with radioactive glucose, noradrenaline causes an increase in the release of radioactivity. These effects were not observed in cultured neuroblastoma cells (Newburg & Rosenburg, 1972). Serotonin was also shown to have a glycogenolytic effect in glial cells. Application of serotonin to the leech segmental ganglia induced a 60% reduction in endogenous glycogen, which occurred in the glial cells of the ganglia (Seal & Pentreath, 1985). Moreover, serotonin, histamine, adenosine, and the structurally related peptides VIP and PHI-27, were found to promote the hydrolysis of [^{3}H]glycogen newly synthesised from [^{3}H]glucose in astroglia cultured from rat brain (Magistretti *et al.*, 1983).

In summary, all these studies indicate that glycogenolysis, in astrocytes, following the conversion of phosphorylase b to a is dependent upon cAMP levels, which in turn are increased by β-adrenergic receptor activation (see Figure 7.3). It appears as if glycogen is a prominent feature of fibrous and protoplasmic astrocytes and retinal glial cells in mammals, though the sub-

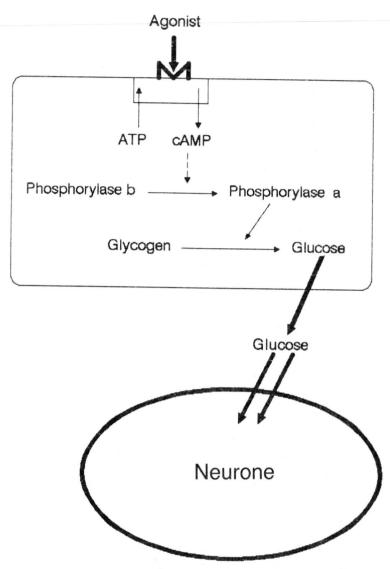

Fig. 7.3   The binding of agonists to glial receptors linked to the production of cAMP may lead to the activation of glycogen phosphorylase (from b to a). Phosphorylase a induces glycogen breakdown thus making glial glucose available for possible use by neurones.

stance exist in lesser amounts in neurones. All the above observations suggest that astrocytes store glycogen for use by neurones. Thus neuroactive substances released when neurones discharge could trigger glycogenolysis in adjacent astrocytes by interacting with the glial receptors and activating adenylate cyclase, making glucose or lactate available for use by neurones. In this manner, the neuronal energy requirements could, to some extent, parallel and be controlled by the degree of neuronal activity.

In support of this, Keller *et al.* (1981) have found that in neuroblastoma cells, steady state intracellular glucose concentrations reached the extracellular levels, while intracellular contents in C6 glioma cells remained very low. Moreover, influx rates of D-glucose in C6 glioma cells were only half those found in neuroblastoma cells. The idea that astrocytic glycogen serves as an energy reserve for neurones in an emergency situation such as hypoglycaemia should not be ignored, since glycogen degradation following the administration of noradrenaline is maximal under conditions where extracellular glucose has been substantially consumed, and minimal under conditions where medium glucose levels are high (Cummins *et al.*, 1983).

7.4 Clinical significance of glial receptors

As mentioned earlier, astrocytes have been shown to take up various substances including GABA, noradrenaline, dopamine and serotonin. The removal of transmitters from the synaptic cleft effectively abolishes continued neurotransmission. The clearance of neurotransmitters from the synapse by glial uptake may, therefore, be a major means by which these cells modulate neurotransmission. In relation to this, various reports have suggested that one of the means by which antidepressants exert their therapeutic action is by inhibition of uptake processes (Iversen, 1965; Carlsson *et al.*, 1969), while others have demonstrated the presence of saturable high affinity binding sites for ^{3}H-imipramine and ^{3}H-mianserin (both antidepressant drugs) in C6 glial cell lines (Whitaker & Warsh, 1983). In primary cultures of astrocytes, it was reported that either long-term treatment with amitriptyline, a tricyclic antidepressant which inhibits noradrenaline and serotonin uptake, or short-term treatment with doxepin, another tricyclic antidepressant, leads to a reduction in isoproterenol-induced accumulation of cAMP (Hertz *et al.*, 1980, 1981). Short-term treatment of astrocytes with the antidepressants tranylcypromine (a monoamine oxidase inhibitor) and amitriptyline had a direct inhibitory effect on the binding of the beta-adrenergic ligand dihydroalprenolol and on the isoproterenol-induced stimulation of cAMP. In contrast, these drugs enhanced the formation of cAMP in the absence of isoproterenol (Hertz & Richardson, 1983). Interestingly, chronic exposure of amitriptyline or tranylcypromine lead to a decrease in isoproterenol-induced accumulation of cAMP in astrocytes (Hertz & Richardson, 1983), and the time course and magnitude of this reduction were found to be comparable to those reported for the down-regulation of β-adrenergic activity in whole brain *in vivo* during chronic exposure to antidepressant drugs (Sulser, 1979).

These findings suggest that antidepressant drugs act as partial agonists at astrocytic β-adrenergic receptors and that the acute interaction is a crucial feature in the mechanism of action of at least some of these drugs. Furthermore, the chronic interaction which leads to down-regulation of β-adrenergic activity in astrocytes may partly explain this phenomenon observed in whole brain evoked by chronic exposure to these drugs. This suggests, in turn, that glial cell abnormalities or malfunctions may be crucially important in the aetiology of affective disorders and perhaps also in other psychiatric illnesses (Henn & Henn, 1980; Hertz, 1982).

7.5 Conclusion

Glial cells play an important role in support of neuronal functions. If glia and neurones are to act as a unit, it is desirable for information to flow from neurones to glia. Substances released from neurones, such as ions, transmitters and catabolic products, are likely to serve as signals to produce a response by the glial cells. These signals may activate any one of the various receptors present on glia, which would eventually modify the extracellular concentration of several neuroactive compounds. Therefore, it seems that neuronal activity and even tonic neuronal secretions have a metabolic autofeedback on neurones themselves. It is clear that glia and neurones are true partners in the nervous system. Further research utilising preparations of isolated glia can be expected to further our current understanding of this critical relationship under both normal and pathological conditions.

Acknowledgement

We are indebted to the wellcome Trust for their support.

7.6 Further reading

(Other literature is listed in the compiled references at the end of the book.)

Berridge, M. J. (1984). Inositol triphosphate and diacylglycerol as second messengers. *Biochemical Journal*, **220**, 345–60.

Cummins, C. J., Lust, W. D. & Passonneau, J. V. (1983). Regulation of glycogenolysis in transformed astrocytes *in vitro*. *Journal of Neurochemistry*, **40**, 137–44.

England, P. J. (1986). Intracellular calcium receptor mechanisms. *British Medical Bulletin*, **42**, 375–83.

Hansson, E. (1986). Primary astroglial cultures: a biochemical and functional evaluation. *Neurochemical Research*, **11**, 759–67.

Henn, F. A. & Henn, S. W. (1980). The psychopharmacology of astroglial cells. *Progress in Neurobiology*, **15**, 1–17.

Hyden, H. (1967). RNA in brain cells. In: *The Neurosciences: a study program*, eds. G. C. Quarton, T. Melnechuck and F. O. Schmitt. Rockefeller University Press, New York.

Kimelberg, H. K. (ed.) (1988). *Glial cell receptors*. Naven Press, New York.

Pearce, B., Cambray-Deakin, M., Morrow, C., Grimble, J. & Murphy, S. (1985a). Activation of muscarinic and of α_1-adrenergic receptors on astrocytes. Results in the accumulation of inositol phosphates. *Journal of Neurochemistry*, **45**, 1534–40.

Pope, A. (1978). Neuroglia: quantitative aspects. In: *Dynamic properties of glia cells*, eds. E. Schoffeniels, G. Frank, L. Hertz & D. B. Tower, pp. 13–20. Pergamon Press, Oxford.

Ramon y Cajal, S. (1928). *Degeneration and regeneration of the nervous system*. Oxford University Press, Oxford.

Van Calker, D. & Hamprecht, B. (1980). Effects of neurohormones on glial cells. In: *Advances in Cellular Neurobiology*, eds. S. Federoff & L. Hertz, pp. 31–67, Academic Press, New York.

Whitaker, P. M. & Warsh, J. J. (1983). Specific binding of radiolabelled antidepressant to brain astroglial cells. In: *CNS Receptors – From Molecular Pharmacology to Behavior*, eds. P. Mandel and F. V. DeFeudis, pp. 477–85. Raven Press, New York.

References

(Other literature is listed in the selected further reading of the end of each chapter.)

Affolter, H., Erne, P., Burgisser, E. & Pletscher, A. (1984). Ca^{2+} as messengers of $5HT_2$-receptor stimulation in human blood plates. *Naunyn-Schmiedeberg's Archives of Pharmacology*, **325**, 337–342.

Agnati, L. F., Fuxe, K., Benfenati, F., Zini, I. & Hokfelt, T. (1983). On the function role of coexistence of 5HT and substance P in bulbospinal 5HT neurons. Substance P reduces affinity and increases density of ^{3}H-5HT binding sites. *Acta Physiologica Scandinavica*, **117**, 299–301.

Andres, R. Y., Rubin, J. S. & Bradshaw, R. A. (1977). Specific nuclear binding of nerve growth factor. *Transactions of the American Society of Neurochemistry*, **8**, 190.

Asada, Y. & Bennett, M. V. L. (1971). Experimental alteration of coupling resistance at an electrotonic synapse. *Journal of Cell Biology*, **49**, 159–72.

Audesirk, G., Audesirk, T. & Bowsher, P. (1982). Variability and frequent failure of Lucifer Yellow to pass between two electrically coupled neurons in *Lymnaea stagnalis*. *Journal of Neurobiology*, **13**, 369–75.

Audigier, S., Barberis, C. & Jard, S. (1986). Vasoactive intestinal polypeptide increases inositol phospholipid breakdown in the rat superior cervical ganglion. *Brain Research*, **378**, 363–7.

Auerbach, A. A. & Bennett M. V. L. (1969). A rectifying synapse in the central nervous system of a vertebrate. *Journal of General Physiology*, **53**, 211–37.

Aurameas, S. (1969). Coupling of enzymes to proteins with glutaraldehyde. Use of conjugates for the detection of antigens and antibodies. *Immunochemistry*, **6**, 43–52.

Azmitia, E. C. (1978). The serotonin producing neuron of the midbrain and dorsal raphe nuclei. In: *Handbook of Pyschopharmacology, 9*, eds. L. L. Iverson, S. D. Iverson, S. H. Snyder, pp. 233–314. Plenum Press, New York.

Balazs, R., Patel, A. J. & Richter, D. (1973). Metabolic compartments in the brain: their properties and relation to morphological structures. In: *Metabolic Compartmentation in the Brain*, eds. R. Balazs & I. E. Cremer, pp. 167–84. The Macmillan Press Ltd., London.

Banerjee, S. P., Snyder, S. H., Cuatrecasas, P. & Greene, L. A. (1973).

Binding of nerve growth factor receptor in sympathetic ganglia. *Proceedings of the National Academy of Sciences, USA*, **70**, 2519–23.

Berry, M. S. and Cottrell, G. A. (1975). Excitatory and inhibitory biphasic synaptic potentials mediated by an identified dopamine-containing neurone. *Journal of Physiology*, **284**, 589–612.

Berry, M. S. and Cottrell, G. A. (1979). Ionic basis of different synaptic potentials mediated by an identified dopamine-containing neurone. *Proceedings of the Royal Society of London, B*, **203**, 427–44.

Barbaccia, M. L., Brunello, N., Chuang, D-M. & Costa, E. (1983). Serotonin elicited amplification of adenylate cyclase activity in hippocampal membranes from adult rat. *Journal of Neurochemistry*, **40**, 1671–9.

Barnstable, C. J. (1980). Monoclonal antibodies which recognize different cell types in the cat retina. *Nature*, **286**, 231–5.

Bass, N. H., Hess, A., Pope, A. & Thalheimer, C. (1971). Quantitative cytoarchitectonic distribution of neurons, glia, and DNA in rat cerebral cortex. *Journal of Comparative Neurology*, **143**, 481–90.

Beattie, M. S., Bresnahn, J. C. & King, J. S. (1978). Ultrastructural identification of dorsal root primary afferent terminals after anterograde filling with horseradish peroxidase. *Brain Research*, **153**, 127–34.

Bentivoglio, M., Kuypers, H. G. J. M. & Catsman-Berrevoets, C. E. (1980a). Retrograde neuronal labelling by means of bisbenzimide and Nuclear Yellow (Hoechst 769121). Measures to prevent diffusion of the tracers out of retrogradely labelled neurones. *Neuroscience Letters*, **18**, 19–24.

Bentivoglio, M., Kuypers, H. G. J. M., Catsman-Berrovoets, C. E., Loewe, H. & Dawn, O. (1980b). Two new fluorescent retrograde tracers which are transported long distances. *Neuroscience Letters*, **18**, 25–30.

Berridge, M. J. (1984). Inositol trisphosphate and diacylglycerol as second messengers. *Biochemical Journal*, **220**, 345–60.

Berridge, M. J. & Irvine, R. F. (1984). Inositol trisphosphate, a novel second messenger in cellular signal transduction. *Nature*, **313**, 315–21.

Birks, R., Katz, B. & Miledi, R. (1960). Physiological and structural changes at the amphibian myoneural junction in the course of nerve degeneration. *Journal Physiology*, **150**, 145–68.

Bito, L. Z., Nichols, R. R. & Baroody, R. A. (1982). A comparison of the miotic and inflammatory effects of biologically active polypeptides and prostaglandin E_2 on the rabbit eye. *Experimental Eye Research*, **34**, 325–37.

Borghi, C., Nicosia, S., Giachetti, A. & Said, S. I. (1979). Vasoactive intestinal polypeptide (VIP) stimulates adenylate cyclase in selected areas of rat brain. *Life Sciences*, **24**, 65–70.

Boyd, I. A. & Martin, A. R. (1956). The end-plate potential in mammalian muscle. *Journal Physiology*, **132**, 74–91.

Bradley, P. B. & Costa, E. (1984). Symposium: 5HT, peripheral and central receptors and function. *Neuropharmacology*, **23**, 1472–569.

Brink, P. & Barr, L. (1977). The resistance of the septum of the median giant axon of the earthworm. *Journal of General Physiology*, **69**, 517–36.

Brostrom, M. A., Brostrom, C. O. & Wolff, D. J. (1979). Calcium dependence of hormone-stimulated cAMP accumulation in intact glial tumour cells. *Journal of Biological Chemistry*, **254**, 7548–57.

Browning, E. T., Schwartz, J. P. & Breckenridge, B. McL. (1974). Norepinephrine-sensitive properties of C-6 astrocytoma cells. *Molecular Pharmacology*, **10**, 162–74.

Burrows, M. (1980). The control of sets of motoneurones by local interneurones in the locust. *Journal of Physiology*, **298**, 213–33.

Cambray-Deakin, M. A., Morrow, C. & Murphy, S. (1985). Cortical astrocytes in primary culture: presence of neurotransmitter binding sites. *Biochemical Society Transactions*, **13**, 231–2.

Carlsson, A., Jonason, J., Lindqvist, M. & Fuxe, K. (1969). Demonstration of extraneuronal 5-hydroxytryptamine accumulation in brain following membrane-pump blockade by chlorimipramine. *Brain Research*, **12**, 456–60.

Castagna, M., Takai, Y., Kaibuchi, K., Sano, K., Kikkawa, U. & Nishizuka, Y. (1982). Direct activation of calcium-activating phospholipid-dependent protein kinase by tumour promoting phrobol esters. *Journal of Biological Chemistry*, **257**, 7847–51.

Ceccarelli, B., Hurlburt, W. P. & Mauro, A. (1972). Depletion of vesicles from frog neuromuscular junctions by prolonged tetanic stimulation. *Journal Cell Biology*, **54**, 30–8.

Chang, M. N. & Leeman, S. E. (1970). Isolation of sialogogi peptide from the bovine hypothalamic tissue & its characterisation as substance P. *Journal of Biological Chemistry*, **245**, 4784–90.

Chan-Palay, V. (1982). Coexistence of traditional neurotransmitters with peptides in the mammalian brain: 5-hydroxytryptamine and substance P in the raphe and gamma aminobutyric acid and motilin in the cerebellum. In: *Cotransmission*, ed. A. C. Cuello, pp. 1–24. Macmillan Press, London.

Changeux, J-P., Devillers-Thiery, A. & Chemouilli, P. (1984). Acetylcholine an allosteric protein. *Science*, **225**, 1335–45.

Childs, G. W. (1986). *Immunocytochemical Technology*. Alan R. Liss, New York.

Clark, A. W., Hurlburt, W. P. & Mauro, A. (1972). Changes in the fine structure of neuromuscular junctions of the frog caused by Black Widow Spider venom. *Journal Cell Biology*, **52**, 1–14.

Clark, R. B. & Perkins, J. P. (1971). Regulation of adenosine 3′:5′-cyclic monophosphate concentration in cultured human astrocytoma cells by catecholamines and histamine. *Proceedings of the National Academy of Sciences USA*, **68**, 2757–60.

Clark, R. B., Su, Y.-F., Ortmann, R., Cubeddu, X., Johnson, G. L. &

Perkins, J. P. (1975). Factors influencing the effect of hormones on the accumulation of cyclic AMP in cultured human astrocytoma cells. *Metabolism*, **24**, 343–58.

Codina, J., Hildebrandt, J., Sunyer, T., Sekura, R. D., Manclark, C. R., Iyengar, R. & Birnbaumer, L. (1984). Mechanisms of vectorial receptor adenylated signal transduction. *Advances in Cyclic Nucleotide Research*, **17**, 111–25.

Cohan, C. S., Hadley, R. D. & Kater, S. B. (1983). 'Zap axotomy': localized fluorescent excitation of single dye-filled neurons induces growth by selective axotomy. *Brain Research*, **270**, 93–101.

Collins, W. F. (1983). Organization of electrical coupling between frog lumbar motoneurons. *Journal of Neurophysiology*, **49**, 730–44.

Conn, P. J. & Sanders-Bush, E. (1984). Selective 5HT-2 antagonists inhibit serotonin stimulated phosphatidyl inositol metabolism in cerebral cortex. *Neuropharmacology*, **23**, 993–6.

Conn, J. P., Sanders-Bush, E., Hoffman B. J. & Hastig P. R. (1986). A unique serotonin receptor in the choroid plexus is linked to phosphatidylinositde turnover. *Proceedings of the National Academy of Sciences, USA*, **83**, 4081–8.

Cook, N. J., Hanke, W. & Kaupp, U. B. (1987). Identification of the cyclic GMP-dependent channel from the rod photoreceptors. *Proceedings of the National Academy of Sciences, USA*, **84**, 585–9.

Coons, A. H. & Kaplan, M. H. (1950). Localization of antigen in tissue cells: II improvements in a method for the detection of antigen by means of fluorescent antibody. *Journal of Experimental Medicine*, **91**, 1–13.

Costa, E., Kurosawa, A. & Guidotti, A. (1976). Activation and nuclear translocation of protein kinase during trans-synaptic induction of tyrosine-3-mono-oxygenase. *Proceedings of the National Academy of Sciences, USA*, **73**, 1058–62.

Cottrell, G. A. (1970). Direct postsynaptic responses to stimulation of serotonin-containing neurones. *Nature*, **225**, 1060–2.

Cottrell, G. A. and Macon, J. B. (1974). Synaptic connexions of two symmetrically placed giant serotonin-containing neurones. *Journal of Physiology*, **236**, 435–64.

Crow, T. J., Cross, A. J., Cooper, S. J., Deakin, J. F. W., Ferrier, I. N., Johnson, J. A., Joseph, M. H., Owen, F., Poulter, M., Lofthouse, R., Corsellis, J. A. N., Chambers, D. R., Blessed, G., Perry, E. K., Perry, R. H. & Tomlinson, B. E. (1984). Neurotransmitter receptors and monoamine metabolites in the brain of patients with Alzheimer type dementia and depression and suicides. *Neuropharmacology*, **23**, 1561–9.

Cuello, A. C. (ed.) (1982). *Cotransmission*, Macmillian Press, London.

Cuello, A. C., Milstein, C. & Priestly, J. V. (1980). Use of monoclonal antibodies in immunochemistry with special reference to the central nervous system. *Brain Research Bulletin*, **5**, 575–87.

Cullheim, S. & Kellerth, J-O. (1976). Combined light and electron microscopic tracing of neurones, including axons and synaptic terminals, after intracellular injection of horseradish peroxidase. *Neuroscience Letters*, **2**, 307–13.

Cutcliffe, N. & Osborne, N. N. (1987). Serotonergic and cholinergic stimulation of inositol phosphate formation in the rabbit retina. Evidence for the presence of 5HT-2 and muscarinic receptors. *Brain Research*. (In press)

Dalsgaard, C-J., Hökfelt, T., Elfvin, L-G., Skirboll, L. & Emson, P. (1982). Substance P-containing primary sensory neurones projecting to the inferior mesenteric ganglion: evidence from combined retrograde tracing and immunochemistry. *Neuroscience*, **7**, 647–54.

Darnell, J., Lodish, H. & Baltimore, D. (1986). *Molecular Cell Biology*. Scientific American Books, New York.

Davis, R. J., Ganong, B. R., Bell, R. M., & Czech, M. P. (1985). Structural requirements for diacylglycerols to mimic tumour promoting phorbol diesterase action on the epidermal growth factor receptor. *Journal of Biological Chemistry*, **260**, 5315–22.

de Courcelles, D. C., Roevens, P. & Van Belle, H. (1984). Stimulation by serotonin of 40 KDa 20 KDa protein phosphorylation in human platelets. *Federation Of European Biochemical Society Letters*, **171**, 289–92.

De Mello, W. C. (1983). The influence of pH on the healing-over of mammalian cardiac muscle. *Journal of Physiology*, **339**, 299–307.

Del Castillo, J. & Katz, B. (1957). La base 'quantale' de la transmission neuro-musculaire. In *Microphysiologie comparée des éléments excitables*. Coll. internat. CNRS, Paris, **67**, 245–58.

Deschodt-Lanckman, M., Roberecht, P. & Christophe, J. (1977). Characterisation of VIP sensitive adenylate cyclase in guinea-pig brain. *Federation of European Society Letters*, **83**, 76–80.

Downes, C. P. (1986). Agonist stimulated phosphatidylinositol 4,5-bisphosphate metabolism in the nervous system. *Neurochemistry International*, **9**, 211–30.

Droz, B. & Leblond, C. P. (1963). Axonal migration of proteins in the central nervous system and peripheral nerves as shown by radioautography. *Journal of Comparative Neurology*, **121**, 325–37.

Dunlap, K., Takeda, K. & Brehm, P. (1987). Activation of a calcium-dependent photoprotein by chemical signalling through gap junctions. *Nature (London)*, **325**, 60–62.

Enevoldson, T. P., Gordon, G. & Sanders, D. J. (1984). The use of retrograde transport of horseradish peroxidase for studying for dendritic trees and axonal courses of particular groups of tract cells in the spinal cord. *Experimental Brain Research*, **54**, 529–37.

Fairén, A., Peters, A. & Saldanha, J. (1977). A new procedure for examining Golgi impregnated neurons by light and electron microscopy. *Journal of Neurocytology*, **6**, 311–37.

Fatt, P. & Katz, B. (1952). Spontaneous subthreshold activity at motor nerve endings. *Journal of Physiology*, **117**, 109–28.

Fesce, R., Grohovaz, F., Hurlburt, W. P. & Ceccarelli, B. (1980). Freeze fracture studies of frog neuromuscular junctions during intense release of neurotransmitter. iii. A morphometric analysis of the number and diameter of intramembrane particles. *Journal of Cell Biology*, **85**, 337–45.

Fillion, G., Roussell, J. C., Beaudoin, D., Pradelles, P., Goiny, M., Dray, F. & Jacob, J. (1979a). Serotonin-sensitive adenylate cyclase in horse brain synaptosomal membranes. *Life Sciences*, **24**, 1813–22.

Fillion, G., Beaudoin, D., Roussell, J. C., Deniau, J. M., Fillion, M. P, Dray, F. & Jacob, J. (1979b). Decrease of ^{3}H-5HT high affinity binding and 5HT adenylate cyclase activation after kainic acid lession in rat brain striatum. *Journal of Neurochemistry*, **33**, 567–70.

Fillion, G., Beaudoin, D., Rousselle, J. C. & Jacob, J. (1980). [^{3}H]5-HT Binding sites and 5-HT-sensitive adenylate cyclase in glial cells membrane fraction. *Brain Research*, **198**, 361–74.

Fillion, G., Beaudoin, D., Fillion, M.-P., Rousselle, J. C., Robaut, C. & Netter, Y. (1983). 5-Hydroxytryptamine receptors in neurones and glia. *Journal of Neural Transmission*, Supplement 18, 307–17.

Finbow, M., Yancey, S. B., Johnson, R., Revel, J.-P. (1980). Independent lines of evidence suggesting a major gap junctional protein with a molecular weight of 26000. *Proceedings of the National Academy of Sciences, USA*, **77**, 970–4.

Finbow, M. E., Shuttleworth, J., Hamilton, A. E. & Pitts, J. D. (1983). Analysis of vertebrate gap junction protein. *EMBO Journal*, **2**, 1479–86.

Fisher, S. K. (1986). Inositol lipid and signal transduction at CNS muscarinic receptors. *Trends In Pharmacology, Supplement: Subtypes of Muscarinic Receptors*, 61–5.

Fisher, S. K. & Bartus, R. T. (1985). Regional differences in the coupling of muscarinic receptors to inositol phospholipid hydrolysis in guinea pig brain. *Journal of Neurochemistry*, **45**, 1085–95.

Flagg-Newton, J. L., Simpson, I. & Loewenstein, W. R. (1979). Permeability of the cell-to-cell membrane channel in mammalian cell junctions. *Science*, **205**, 404–7.

Flink, R. & Westman, J. (1985). Convergence of the same neurons in the feline ventrobasal thalamus of terminals from the dorsal column and the lateral cervical nuclei: an ultra-structural study combining orthograde degeneration and anterograde transport of lectin-conjugated horseradish peroxidase. *Neuroscience Letters*, **61**, 243–8.

Forssmann, W-G., Pickel, V., Reinecke, M., Hock., D. & Metz, J. (1981). Immunohistochemistry and immunocytochemistry of nervous tissue. In: *Techniques in neuroanatomical research*, eds. Ch. Heym & W-G. Forssmann, pp. 171–205. Springer-Verlag, Berlin, Heidelberg, New York.

Frazier, W. A., Boyd, L. F. & Bradshaw, R. A. (1974). Properties of the specific binding of ^{125}I-nerve growth factor to responsive peripheral neurons. *Journal of Biological Chemistry*, **249**, 5513–9.

Freund, T. F. & Somogyi, P. (1983). The section–Golgi impregnation procedure. 1. Description of the method and its combination with histochemistry after intracellular iontophoresis or retrograde transport of horseradish peroxidase. *Neuroscience*, **9**, 463–74.

Freund, T. F., Powell, J. F. & Smith, A. D. (1984). Tyrosine hydroxylase-immunoreactive boutons in synaptic contact with identified striatonigral neurones, with particular reference to dendritic spines. *Neuroscience*, **13**, 1189–215.

Furshpan, E. J. & Potter, D. D. (1959). Transmission at the giant motor synapses of the crayfish. *Journal of Physiology*, **145**, 289–325.

Gardner, D. and Kandel, E. R. (1972). Diphasic postsynaptic potential: a chemical synapse capable of mediating conjoint excitation and inhibition. *Science*, **173**, 550–3.

Gerfen, C. R. & Sawchenko, P. E. (1984). An anterograde neuroanatomical tracing method that shows the detailed morphology of neurons, their axons and terminals: immunohistochemical localization of an axonally transported plant lectin, *Phaseolus vulgaris* leucoagglutinin (PHA-L). *Brain Research*, **290**, 219–38.

Gerfen, G. D., O'Leary, D. D. M. & Cowan, W. M. (1982). A note on the transneuronal transport of wheatgerm agglutinin-conjugated horseradish peroxidase in the avian and rodent visual systems. *Experimental Brain Research*, **48**, 443–8.

Gerschenfeld, H. M. and Paupardin-Tritsch, D. (1974). On the transmitter function of 5-hydroxytryptamine at excitatory and inhibitory monosynaptic junctions. *Journal of Physiology*, **243**, 457–81.

Ghazi, H. & Osborne, N. (1988). Agonist-induced stimulation of inositol phosphates in primary rabbit retinal cultures. *Journal of Neurochemistry*, **50**, 1851–8.

Giaume, C. & Korn, H. (1983). Bidirectional transmission at the rectifying electrotonic synapse: a voltage-dependent process. *Science*, **220**, 84–7.

Giaume, C. & Korn, H. (1984). Voltage-dependent dye coupling at the rectifying electrotonic synapse of the crayfish. *Journal of Physiology*, **356**, 151–67.

Giaume, C., Spira, M. E. & Korn, H. (1980). Uncoupling of invertebrate electrotonic synapses by carbon dioxide. *Neuroscience Letters*, **17**, 197–202.

Gil, D. W. & Wolfe, B. B. (1985). Pirenzepine distinguishes between muscarinic receptor-mediated phosphoinositol breakdown and inhibition of adenylate cyclase. *Journal of Pharmacology and Experimental Therapeutics*, **232**, 608–16.

Gilbert, R. F. T., Emson, P. C., Hunt, S. P., Bennett, G. W., Marsden, C. A., Sandberg, B. E. B., Steinbusch, H. & Verfiofstad, A. A. J. (1982). The effects of monoamine neurotoxins on peptides in the rat spinal cord. *Neuroscience*, **7**, 69–88.

Gillette, R. & Pomeranz, B. (1973). Neuron geometry and circuitry via electron microscope: intracellular staining with osmiophillic polymer. *Science*, **182**, 1256–8.

Gilman, A. G. & Nirenberg, M. (1971). Effect of catecholamine on the adenosine 3':5'-cyclic monophosphate concentrations of clonal satellite cells of neurons. *Proceedings of the National Academy of Sciences, USA*, **68**, 2167–8.

Gilman, A. G. (1972). Regulation of cyclic AMP metabolism in cultured cells of the nervous system. *Advances in Cyclic Nucleotide Research*, **1**, 489–510.

Gilman, A. G. & Schrier, B. K. (1972). Adenosine cyclic 3',5'-monophosphate in fetal rat brain cell cultures I. Effects of catecholamines. *Molecular Pharmacology*, **8**, 410–6.

Goldberg, S. & Kotani, M. (1967). The projection of the optic nerve fibres in the frog *Rana catesbeiana* as studied by radioautography. *Anatomical Record*, **158**, 325–32.

Goodenough, D. A. (1974). Bulk isolation of mouse hepatocyte gap junctions. Characterization of the principal protein. Connexin. *Journal of Cell Biology*, **61**, 557–63.

Gonatas, N. K., Harper, C., Mizutani, T. & Gonatas, J. O. (1979). Superior sensitivity of conjugates of horseradish peroxidase with wheat-germ agglutinin for studies in retrograde axonal transport. *Journal of Histochemistry and Cytochemistry*, **27**, 728–34.

Grafstein, B. (1971). Transneuronal transfer of radioactivity in the central nervous system. *Science*, **172**, 177–9.

Graham, R. C. & Karnowsky, M. J. (1966). The early stages of absorption of horseradish peroxidase into the proximal tubules of mouse kidney: ultrastructural cytochemistry by a new technique. *Journal of Histochemistry and Cytochemistry*, **14**, 291–302.

Grant, G., Arvidsson, J., Robertson, B. & Ygge, J. (1979). Transganglionic transport of horseradish peroxidase in primary sensory neurones. *Neuroscience Letters*, **12**, 23–8.

Graubard, K., Raper, J. A. & Hartline, D. K. (1983). Graded synaptic transmission between identified spiking neurones. *Journal of Neurophysiology*, 50, 508–21.

Gray, E. G. (1975). Synaptic fine structure and nuclear cytoplasmic and extracellular networks. The stereoframework concept. *Journal Neurocytology*, **4**, 315–39.

Groenwegen, H. J. & van Dijk, C. A. (1984). Efferent connections of the dorsal tegmental region in the rat. Studied by means of anterograde transport of the lectin *Phaseolus vulgaris* – leucoagglutinin (PHA-L). *Brain Research*, **304**, 367–71.

Guth, L. & Watson, P. K. (1968). A correlated histochemical and quantitative study on cerebral glycogen after brain injury in the rat. *Experimental Neurology*, **22**, 590–602.

Hadley, R. D., Wong, R. G., Kater, S. B., Barker, D. L. & Bulloch, A. G. M. (1982). Formation of novel central and peripheral connections between molluscan central neurons in organ cultured ganglia. *Journal of Neurobiology*, **13**, 217–30.

Hamberger, A. & Hyden, H. (1963). Inverse enzymatic changes in neurons and glia during increased function and hypoxia. *Journal of Cell Biology*, **16**, 521–5.

Hamberger, A., Blomstrand, C. & Lehninger, A. (1970). Comparative studies on mitochondria isolated from neuron-enriched and glia-enriched fractions of rabbit and beef brain. *Journal of Cell Biology*, **45**, 221–34.

Hammer, R. & Giachetti, A. (1982). Muscarinic receptor subtypes: M1 and M2. Biochemical and functional characterisation. *Life Sciences*, **31**, 2991–8.

Hanker, J. S., Yates, P. E., Metz, C. & Rustioni, A. (1977). A new specific, sensitive and non-carcinogenic reagent for the demonstration of horseradish peroxidase. *Histochemical Journal*, **9**, 789–92.

Hanna, R. B., Keeter, J. S. & Pappas, G. D. (1978). The fine structure of a rectifying electrotonic synapse. *Journal of Cell Biology*, **79**, 764–73.

Hansson, E., Ronnback, L. & Sellstrom, A. (1984). Is there a 'dopaminergic glial cell'? *Neurochemical Research*, **9**, 679–89.

Harrison, P. J., Hultborn, H. Jankowska, E., Katz, R., Storai, B., & Zytnicki, D. (1984). Labelling of interneurones by retrograde trans-synaptic transport of horseradish peroxidase from motoneurones in rats and cats. *Neuroscience Letters*, **45**, 15–19.

Haydon, P. G. (1989). Formation of chemical synapses: neuronal strategies. In *The Cellular Basis of Neuronal Plasticity: Physiology, Morphology and Biochemistry of Molluscan Neurones*, ed. A. G. M. Bulloch, pp. 129–51. Manchester University Press, Manchester, UK.

Heitler, W. J., Cobb, J. L. S. & Fraser, K. (1985). Ultrastructure of the segmental giant neuron of crayfish. *Journal of Neurocytology*, **14**, 921–41.

Hendrickson, A. E. (1972). Electron microscopic distribution of axoplasmic transport. *Journal of Comparative Neurology*, **144**, 381–98.

Hendry, I. A., Stoeckel, K., Thoenen, H. & Iversen, L. (1974). The retrograde axonal transport of nerve growth factor. *Brain Research*, **68**, 103–21.

Henn, F. A., Anderson, D. J. and Sellstrom, A. (1977). Possible relationship between glial cells, dopamine and the effects of antipsychotic drugs. *Nature*, **266**, 637–8.

Hertz, L., Baldwin, F. & Schousboe, A. (1979). Serotonin receptors on astrocytes in primary cultures: effects of methysergide and fluoxetine. *Canadian Journal of Physiology Pharmacology*, **57**, 223–6.

Hertz, L., Richardson, J. S. & Mukerji, S. (1980). Doxepin, a tricyclic antidepressant, binds to normal, intact astroglial cells in cultures and inhibits the isoproterenol-induced increase in cyclic AMP production. *Canadian Journal of Physiology Pharmacology*, **58**, 1515–9.

Hertz, L., Mukerji, S. & Richarson, J. S. (1981). Down-regulation of beta-adrenergic activity in astroglia by chronic treatment with antidepressant drug. *European Journal of Pharmacology*, **72**, 267–8.

Hertz, L. (1982). Astrocytes. In: *Handbook of Neurochemistry*, ed. A. Lajtha, pp. 319–55. Plenum Press, New York.

Hertz, L. & Richardson, J. S. (1983). Acute and chronic effects of antidepressant drugs on beta-adrenergic function in astrocytes in primary cultures: An indication of glial involvement in affective disorders? *Journal of Neuroscience Research*, **9**, 173–82.

Hertzberg, E. L. & Gilula, N. B. (1979). Isolation and characterization of gap junctions from rat liver. *Journal of Biological Chemistry*, **254**, 2138–47.

Hertzberg, E. L. (1985). Antibody probes in the study of gap junctional communication. *Annual Review of Physiology*, **47**, 305–18.

Heuser, J. E. & Reese, T. S. (1973). Evidence for recycling of synaptic vesicle membrane during transmitter release at the frog neuromuscular junction. *Journal of Cell Biology*, **57**, 315–44.

Heuser, J. E. & Reese, T. S. (1981). Structural changes after transmitter release at the frog neuromuscular junction. *Journal of Cell Biology*, **88**, 564–80.

Heuser, J. E., Katz, B. & Miledi, R. (1971). Structural and functional changes of frog neuromuscular junctions in high calcium solutions. *Proceedings of the Royal Society of London, B*, **178**, 407–15.

Heuser, J. E., Reese, T. S., Dennis, M., Jan, Y., Jan, L. & Evans, L. (1979). Synaptic vesicle exocytosis captured by quick freezing and correlated with quantal transmitter release. *Journal of Cell Biology*, **81**, 275–300.

Hirata, H., Slater, N. T. & Kimelberg, H. K. (1983). Alpha-adrenergic receptor-mediated depolarization of rat neocortical astrocytes in primary culture. *Brain Research*, **270**, 358–62.

Hokin L. E. & Hokin M. R. (1955). Effects of acetylcholine on the turnover of phosphoryl units in individual phospholipids of pancreas slices and brain cortex. *Biochemica Biophysica Acta*, **18**, 102–10.

Holzer, P. & Lippe, I. T. (1985). Substance P action on phosphoinositides in guinea pig intestinal muscle: a possible transduction mechanism? *Naunyn-Schmiedeberg's Archives of Pharmacology*, **329**, 50–5.

Hosli, E. & Hosli, L. (1982). Evidence for the existence of alpha- and beta- adrenoceptors on neurones and glial cells of cultured rat central nervous system – an autoradiographic study. *Neuroscience*, **7**, 2873–81.

Hosli, E. & Hosli, L. (1984). Autoradiographic localization of binding sites for [^{3}H]histamine and H_1- and H_2-antagonists on cultured neurones and glial cells, *Neuroscience*, **13**, 863–70.

Hosli, L., Hosli, E., Schneider, U. & Wiget, W. (1984). Evidence for the existence of histamine H_1- and H_2-receptors on astrocytes of cultured rat central nervous system. *Neuroscience Letters*, **48**, 287–91.

Hosli, L., Hosli, E., Zehntner, C., Lehmann, R. & Lutz, W. (1982). Evidence for the existence of alpha- and beta-adrenoceptors on cultured glial cells – an electrophysiological study. *Neuroscience*, 7, 2867–72.

Houchin, R. J. Maxwell, D. J., Fyffe, R. E. W. & Brown, A. G. (1983). Light and electron microscopy of dorsal spinocerebellar tract neurones in the cat: an intracellular horseradish peroxidase study. *Quarterly Journal of Experimental Physiology*, 68, 719–32.

Hsu, S-M., Raine, L. & Fanger, H. (1981). Use of avidin–biotin–peroxidase complex (ABC) in inmmunoperoxidase techniques. *Journal of Histochemistry and Cytochemistry*, 29, 577–80.

Huganir, R. L, Albert, K. A. & Greengard, P. (1983). Phosphorylation of the nicotinic acetylcholine receptor by Ca^{2+} phospholipid-dependent protein kinase and comparison with its phosporylation by cAMP-dependent protein kinase. *Society of Neuroscience Abstracts*, 9, 578.

Huganir, R. L. & Greengard, P. (1983). cAMP-dependent protein kinase phosphorylates nicotinic acetylcholine receptor. *Proceedings of the National Academy of Sciences, USA*, 80, 1130–4.

Hughes, A. R, Martin, M. W. & Harden, T. K. (1984). Pertussis toxin differentiates between two mechanisms of attenuation of cyclic AMP accumulation by muscarinic cholinergic receptors. *Proceedings of the National Academy of Sciences, USA*, 80, 5680–4.

Hyden, H. (1962). Cytophysiological aspects of the nucleic acids and proteins of nervous tissue. In: *Neurochemistry*, eds. K. A. C. Elliot, I. H. Page & J. H. Quastel, pp. 331–75. Thomas, Springfield, Illinois.

Hyden, H. & Lange, P. W. (1962). A kinetic study of the neuron–glia relationship. *Journal of Cell Biology*, 13, 233–7.

Itaya, S. K. & van Hoesen, G. W. (1982). WGA–HRP as a transneuronal marker in the visual pathways of monkey and rat. *Brain Research*, 236, 199–204.

Iversen, L. L. (1965). Inhibition of noradrenaline uptake by drugs. *Journal of Pharmacological Pharmacology*, 17, 62–4.

Iversen, L. L. & Bloom, F. E. (1970). Transmitter release mechanisms. *Neuroscience Research Program Bulletin*, 8, 407–20.

Jacob, S., Sahyoun, N. E., Saltiel. A. R. & Cuatrecasas, P. (1983). Phorbol esters stimulate the phosphorylation of receptors for insulin and somatomedin C. *Proceedings of the National Academy of Sciences, USA*, 80, 6211–3.

Jankowska, E. & Lindström, S. (1970). Morphological identification of physiologically defined neurones in the cat spinal cord. *Brain Research*, 20, 323–6.

Jankowska, E., Rastad, J. & Westman, J. (1976). Intracellular application of horseradish peroxidase and its light and electron microscopical appearance in spinocervical tract cells. *Brain Research*, 105, 557–62.

Jard, S., Premont, J. & Benda, P. (1972). Adenylate cyclase phosphodiesterases and protein kinase of rat glial cells in culture. *Federation of European Biochemical Societies Letters*, **26**, 344–8.

Johnston, M. F. & Ramon, F. (1982). Electrotonic coupling in internally perfused crayfish segmented axons. *Journal of Physiology*, **317**, 509–18.

Kandel, E. R., Frazier, W. T., Waziri, R. and Coggeshall, R. E. (1967). Direct and common connections among identified neurons in *Aplysia*. *Journal of Neurophysiology*, **30**, 1352–76.

Kasa, P., Vanyai, E., Farkas, Z. & Pakaski, M. (1984). Choline mobilization from glial cells by stimulation of their muscarinic receptors. In: *Regulation of transmitter function*, eds. E. S. Vizi & K. Magyar, pp. 487–8. Elsevier, Amsterdam.

Keller, K., Lange, K. & Noske, W. (1981). D-Glucose transport in cultured cells of neural origin: The membrane as possible control point of glucose utilization. *Journal of Neurochemistry*, **36**, 1012–7.

Kendall, D. A. & Nahorski, S. R. (1984). Inositol phospholipid hydrolysis in rat brain cerebral cortex slcies II: Calcium requirements. *Journal of Neurochemistry*, **42**, 1388–94.

Kitai, S. T., Kocsis, J. D., Preston, R. J. & Sugimori, M. (1976). Monosynaptic inputs to caudate neurons identified by intracellular injection of horseradish peroxidase. *Brain Research*, **109**, 601–6.

Klee, W. A, Koski, G., Tocque, B. & Simonds, W. F. (1984). On the mechanism of receptor-mediated inhibition of adenylate cyclase. *Advances in Cyclic Nucleotide Research*, **17**, 153–9.

Klein, R. L., Lagercrantz, H. & Zimmermann, H. (1982). *Neurotransmitter Vesicles*. Academic Press, London.

Koh, S.-W., Kyristsis, A. & Chader, G. J. (1984). Interaction of neuropeptides and cultured glial (Muller) cell of the chick retina: Elevation of intracellular cyclic AMP by vasoactive intestinal peptide and glucagon. *Journal of Neurochemistry*, **43**, 199–203.

Köhler, G. & Milstein, C. (1975). Continuous cultures of fused cells secreting antibody of predefined specificity. *Nature*, **256**, 495–7.

Korr, H. (1981). Light microscopical autoradiography of Nervous tissue. In: Techniques in Neuroanatomical Research, eds. Ch. Heym & W-G. Forssmann, Springer-Verlag, Berlin, Heidelberg, New York.

Kriebel, M. E., Bennet, M. V. L., Waxman, S. G. & Pappas, G. D. (1969). Oculomotor neurons in fish: electrotonic coupling and multiple sites of impulse initiation. *Science*, **166**, 520–4.

Krieger, D. T. (1983). Brain peptides what where & why? *Science*, **222**, 975–85.

Kuffler, S. W.,Nicholls, J. G. & Martin, A. R. (1984). *From Neuron to Brain*. Sinauer Associates, Sunderland, MA.

Kuypers, H. G. J. M., Bentivoglio, M., van der Kooy, D. & Catsman-Berrevoets. (1979). Retrograde transport of bisbenzimide and propidium iodide through axons to their parent cell bodies. *Neuroscience Letters*, **12**, 1–7.

Kuypers, H. G. J. M., Bentivoglio, M., Catsman-Berrevoets, C. E. & Bharos, A. T. (1980). Double retrograde neuronal labelling through divergent axon collaterals using two fluorescent tracers with the same excitation wavelength which label different features of the cell. *Experimental Brain Research*, **40**, 383–92.

Lasater, E. M. & Dowling, J. E. (1985). Electrical coupling between pairs of isolated fish horizontal cells is modulated by dopamine and cAMP. In: *Gap Junctions*, eds. M. V. L. Bennett & D. C. Spray, pp. 393–404, Cold Spring Harbor Laboratory.

La Vail, J. H. & La Vail, M. M. (1974). The retrograde intraaxonal transport of horseradish peroxidase in the chick visual system: a light and electron microscopic study. *Journal of Comparative Neurology*, **157**, 303–58.

Le Vay, S. & Gilbert, C. D. (1976). Laminar projections of geniculocortical projection in the cat. *Brain Research*, **113**, 1–19.

Levine, R. R. Birdsall N. J. M., Giachetti, A., Hammer, R., Iverson, L. L., Jenden, D. J. & North R. A. (eds.) (1985). Subtypes of muscarinic receptors II. *Trends in Pharmacological Sciences*, Supplement.

Levitan, H. and Tauc, L. (1972). Acetylcholine receptors: topographic distribution and pharmacological properties of two receptor types on a single molluscan neurone. *Journal of Physiology*, **222**, 537–58.

Leysen, J. E, De Chaffoy, D-C., De Clerck, F., Niemegeers, C. J. E. & Van Nueten, J. M. (1984). Serotonin-S$_2$ receptor binding sites and functional correlations. *Neuropharmacology*, **23**, 1493–501.

Light, A. R. & Durcovic, R. G. (1976). Horseradish peroxidase: an improvement in intracellular staining of single, electrophysiologically characterized neurons. *Experimental Neurology*, **53**, 847–53.

Lincoln, T. M & Corbin, (1983). Characterisation and biological role of cyclic GMP-dependent protein kinase. *Advances in Cyclic Nucleotide Research*, **15**, 139–92.

Llinas, R., Blinks, J. R. & Nicholson, C. (1972). Calcium transient in presynaptic terminal of squid giant synapse: detection with aequorin. *Science*, **176**, 1127–9.

Lundberg, J. M. (1981). Evidence of coexistence of vasoactive intestinal polypeptide (VIP) and acetylcholine in neurons of cat exocrine glands. *Acta Physiologica Scandinavica*, Supplement, **496**, 1–57.

Lundberg, J. M. (1982). Vasoactive intestinal polypeptide enhances muscarinic ligand binding in cat submandibular gland. *Nature*, **295**, 147–9.

Lundberg, J. M. & Hökflet, T. (1983). Coexistence of peptides and classical neurotransmitters. *Trends in Neurosciences*, **6**, 325–33.

Lynch, G., Smith, R. L., Mernsah, P. & Cotman, C. (1973). Tracing the dentate gyrus mossy fibre system with horseradish peroxidase histochemistry. *Experimental Neurology*, **40**, 516–24.

McCarthy, K. D. & deVellis, J. (1978). Alpha-adrenergic receptor modulation of beta-adrenergic, adenosine and prostaglandin E$_1$ increased adenosine 3':5'-monophosphate levels in primary cultures of glia. *Journal of Cyclic Nucleotide Research*, **4**, 15–26.

Magistretti, P. J., Manthorpe, M., Bloom, F. E. & Varon, S. (1983). Functional receptors for vasoactive intestinal polypeptide in cultured astroglia from neonatal rat brain. *Regulatory Peptides*, **6**, 71–80.

Makowski, L., Caspar, D. L. D., Phillips, W. C. & Goodenough, D. A. (1977). Gap junction structures. II. Analysis of the X-ray diffraction data. *Journal of Cell Biology*, **74**, 629–45.

Makowski, L., Caspar, D. L. D., Phillips, W. C. & Baker, T. S. (1984). Gap junction structure. VI. Variation and conservation in connexon conformation and packing. *Biophysics Journal*, **45**, 208–18.

Mallat, M. E. & Hamon, M. (1982). Ca^{2+}-guanine nucleotide interactions in brain membranes. I Modulation of central 5-hydroxytryptamine receptors in the rat. *Journal of Neurochemistry*, **38**, 151–61.

Maranto, A. R. (1982). A photo-oxidation reaction makes Lucifer Yellow useful for electron microscopy. *Science*, **217**, 953–5.

Martin, A. R. (1977). Junctional transmission. ii. Presynaptic mechanisms. In *Handbook of Physiology*, section 1: *The Nervous System*, vol. 1, ed. E. R. Kandel, pp. 329–56. American Physiological Society, Bethesda, MD.

Masters, S. B., Harden, T. K. & Brown, J. H. (1984). Relationships between phosphoinositide and calcium responses to muscarinic agonists in astrocytoma cells. *Molecular Pharmacology*, **26**, 149–55.

Matthews, G. (1987). Single channel recordings demonstrate that cGMP opens the light-sensitive ion channels of the rod photoreceptor. *Proceedings of the National Academy of Sciences, USA*, **84**, 299–302.

Maxwell, D. J. (1985). Combined light and electron microscopy of Golgi-labelled neurons of lamina III of the spinal cord. *Journal of Anatomy*, **141**, 155–69.

Maxwell, D. J., Fyffe, R. E. W. & Brown, A. G. (1984a). Fine structure of normal and degenerating primary afferent boutons associated with characterized spinocervical tract neurones in the cat. *Neuroscience*, **12**, 151–63.

Maxwell, D. J., Bannatyne, B. A., Fyffe, R. E. W. & Brown, A. G. (1984b). Fine structure of primary afferent axon terminals projecting from rapidly adapting mechanoreceptors of the toe and foot pads of the cat. *Quarterly Journal of Experimental Physiology*, **69**, 381–92.

Maxwell, D. J., Koerber, H. R. & Bannatyne, B. A. (1985). Light and electron microscopy of contacts between primary afferent fibres and neurones ascending the dorsal columns of the feline spinal cord. *Neuroscience*, **16**, 375–95.

Mesulam, M-M, (1978). Tetramethyl benzidine for horseradish peroxidase neurohistochemistry: a non-carcinogenic blue reaction product with superior sensitivity for visualizing neural afferents and efferents. *Journal of Histochemistry and Cytochemistry*, **26**, 106–17.

Mesulam, M-M. & Brushart, T. M. (1979). Transganglionic and anterograde transport of horseradish peroxidase across dorsal root ganglia: a tetramethyl benzidine method for tracing central sensory connections of muscles and peripheral nerves. *Neuroscience*, **4**, 1107–17.

Mesulam, M-M. & Mufson, E. J. (1980). The rapid anterograde transport of horseradish peroxidase. *Neuroscience*, **5**, 1277–86.

Metz, C. B., Kavookjain, A. M. & Light, A. R. (1983). Techniques for HRP intracellular staining of neuronal elements for light and electron microscopical analysis. *Journal of Electrophysiological Techniques*, **9**, 151–63.

Miledi, R. & Slater, C. R. (1968). Electrophysiology and electron-microscopy of rat neuromuscular junctions after nerve degeneration. *Proceedings of the Royal Society of London*, B, **169**, 280–306.

Miledi, R. & Slater, C. R. (1970). On the degeneration of rat neuromuscular junctions after nerve section. *Journal of Physiology*, **207**, 507–28.

Mishina, M., Tobimasa, T., Imoto, K., Tanaka, K., Fujita, Y., Fukuda, M., Kurasaki, M., Takahashi, H., Morimoto, Y., Hirose, T., Inayama, S., Takahashi, T., Kuno, M. & Numa, S. (1985). Location of functional regions of acetylcholine receptor alpha-subunits by site directed mutagensis. *Nature*, **313**, 364–9.

Mittag, T. W. & Tormay, A. (1985). Drug responses of adenylate cyclase in iris–ciliary body determined by adenine labelling. *Investigative Ophthalmology and Visual Sciences*, **26**, 396–9.

Muller, K. J. & McMahan, U. J. (1976). The shapes of sensory motor neurons and the distribution of synapses in the ganglia of the leech: A study using intracellular injection of horseradish peroxidase: *Proceedings of the Royal Society of London, B*, **194**, 481–99.

Murphy, A. D., Hadley, R. D. & Kater, S. B. (1983). Axotomy-induced parallel increases in electrical and dye coupling between identified neurons of *Helisoma*. *Journal of Neuroscience*, **3**, 1422–29.

Nagata, Y., Mikoshiba, K. & Tsukada, Y. (1974). Neuronal cell body enriched and glial cell enriched fractions from young and adult rat brains: Preparation and morphological and biochemical properties. *Journal of Neurochemistry*, **22**, 493–503.

Nairn, A. C., Hemmings, H. C. & Greengard, P. (1985). Protein kinases in the brain. *Annual Review of Biochemistry*, **54**, 931–76.

Newburgh, R. W. & Rosenburg, R. N. (1972). Effect of norepinephrine on glucose metabolism in glioblastoma and neuroblastoma cells in cell culture. *Proceedings of the National Academy of Sciences, USA*, **69**, 1677–80.

Nicholson, B. J., Takemoto, L. J., Hunkapiller, M. W., Hood, L. E. & Revel, J.-P. (1983). Differences between the liver gap junction protein and lens MIP26 from rat: Implications for tissue specificity of gap junctions. *Cell*, **32**, 967–78.

Obaid, A. L., Socolar, S. J. & Rose, B. (1983). Cell-to-cell channels with two independent regulated gates in series: analysis of junctional channel modulation by membrane potential, calcium and pH. *Journal of Membrane Biology*, **73**, 69–89.

Okamoto, M., Longenecker, H. E., Riker, W. F. & Song, S. K. (1971). Destruction of mammalian motor nerve terminals by Black Widow Spider venom. *Science*, **172**, 733–6.

Oldfield, B. J. & McLachlan, E. M. (1977). Uptake and retrograde transport of horseradish peroxidase by axons of intact and damaged peripheral nerve trunks. *Neuroscience Letters*, **6**, 135–41.

Olianas, M. C., Onali, P., Nef, N. H. & Costa, E. (1983a). Muscarinic receptors modulate dopamine-activated adenylate cyclase of the rat striatum. *Journal of Neurochemistry*, **41**, 1364–9.

Olianas, M. C., Onali, P., Nef, N. H. & Costa, E. (1983b). Adenylate cyclase activity of synaptic membranes from rat striatum. *Molecular Pharmacology*, **23**, 393–8.

Opler, L. A. & Makman, M. H. (1972). Mediation by cyclic AMP of hormone-stimulated glycogenolysis in cultured rat astrocytoma. *Biochemical and Biophysical Research Communications*, **46**, 1140–5.

Osborne, N. N. (1980). Communication between neurones: Current concepts. *Neurochemistry International*, **3**, 1–6.

Osborne, N. N. (ed.) (1982a). *Biology of serotonergic transmission.* Wiley, Chichester.

O'Shea, M. & Rowell, C. H. F. (1975). A spike-transmitting electrical synapse between visual interneurons in the locust movement detector system. *Journal of Comparative Physiology*, **97**, 143–58.

Palade, G. E. (1954). Electron microscope observations of interneuronal and neuromuscular synapses. *Anatomical Record*, **118**, 336.

Palay, S. L. (1954). Electron microscope study of the cytoplasm of neurons. *Anatomical Record*, **118**, 336.

Passonneau, J. V. & Lowry, O. H. (1971). Metabolite influx in single neurons during ischemia and anesthesia. In: *Recent Advances in Histo- and Cytochemistry*, eds. U. C. Dubach & U. Schmidt, pp. 62–83. Hans Huber Publisher, Bern.

Passonneau, J. V. & Crites, S. K. (1976). Regulation of glycogen metabolism in astrocytoma and neuroblastoma cells in culture. *Journal of Biological Chemistry*, **251**, 2051–22.

Payton, B. W., Bennett, M. V. L. & Pappas, G. D. (1969). Permeability and structure of junctional membranes at an electrical synapse. *Science*, **166**, 1641–3.

Pearce, B. R., Cambray-Deakin, M. A. & Murphy, S. (1985b). Glial glycogen stores are regulated by alpha-adrenergic receptors. *Biochemical Society Transactions*, **13**, 232–3.

Pediga, N. W., Yamamura, H. I. & Nelson, D. L. (1981). Discrimination of multiple ^{3}H-5-hydroxytryptamine binding sites by the neuroleptic spiperone in rat brain. *Journal of Neurochemistry*, **36**, 220–6.

Pelletier, G., Steinbusch, H. W. M. & Verhofstad, A. A. J. (1981).

Immunoreactive substance P and serotonin present in the same dense core vesicles. *Nature*, **293**, 71–2.

Peracchia, C. (1973a). Low resistance junctions in crayfish. I. Two arrays of globules in junctional membranes. *Journal of Cell Biology*, **57**, 54–65.

Peracchia, C. (1973b). Low resistance junctions in crayfish. II. Structural details and further evidence for intercellular channels by freeze-fracture and negative staining. *Journal of Cell Biology*, **57**, 66–76.

Peroutka, S. J., Lebovitz, R. M. & Snyder, S. H. (1979). Serotonin receptor binding affected differentially by guanine nucleotides. *Molecular Pharmacology*, **16**, 700–8.

Peroutka, S. J. & Snyder, S. H. (1979). Multiple serotonin receptors: Differential binding of ^{3}H-serotonin, ^{3}H-lysergic acid diethylamide and ^{3}H-spiperidol. *Molecular Pharmacology*, **16**, 687–99.

Polak, J. M. & van Noorden, S. (1983). *Immunocytochemistry: Practical Applications in Pathology and Biology*. Wright PSG, Bristol, London, Boston.

Polak, J. M. & Varndell, I. M. (1984). *Immunolabelling for Electron Microscopy*. Elsevier, Amsterdam, New York, Oxford.

Powell, S. L. & Westerfield, M. (1984). The absence of specific dye-coupling among frog spinal neurons. *Brain Research*, **294**, 9–14.

Preston, R. J., Bishop, G. A. & Kitai, S. T. (1980). Medium spiny projections from the rat striatum: an intracellular horse-radish peroxidase study. *Brain Research*, **183**, 253–63.

Probert, L., De Mey, J. & Polak, J. M. (1981). Distinct subpopulations of enteric P-type neurones contain substance P and vasoactive intestinal polypeptide. *Nature*, **294**, 470–1.

Proshansky, E. & Egger, M. D. (1977). Staining of the dorsal root projections to the cat's dorsal horn by anterograde movement of horseradish peroxidase. *Neuroscience Letters*, **5**, 103–10.

Purves, D. & McMahan, U. J. (1972). The distribution of synapses on a physiologically identified motor neuron in the central nervous system of the leech. *Journal of Cell Biology*, **55**, 205–20.

Pysh, J. J. & Wiley, R. G. (1972). Morphological alterations of synapses in electrically stimulated superior cervical ganglia of the cat. *Science*, **176**, 191–3.

Quik, M., Iversen, L. L. & Bloom, S. R. (1978). Effects of vasoactive intestinal peptide (VIP) and other peptides on cAMP accumulation in rat brain. *Biochemical Pharmacology*, **27**, 2209–13.

Raese, J. D., Mark, G. & Barchas, J. D. (1981). Regulatory properties of tyrosine hydroxylase multiple froms, subunit structure and cyclic nucleotide independent phosphorylation. In: *Function and regulation of monoamine enzymes. Basic and clinical aspects*, eds. E. Usdin, N. Weiner & M. B. H. Youbim, pp. 105–14. Macmillan Press, New York.

Ramon, F., Zampighi, G. A. & Rivera, A. (1985). Control of junctional permeability. In: *Gap Junctions*, eds. M. V. L. Bennett & D. C. Spray, pp. 155–166. Cold Spring Harbor Laboratory.

Rapava, E. A., Kuz'mina, S. N. & Zbarskii, I. B. (1973). Oxidative phosphorylation and ATPase activity of isolated nuclei and nuclear envelopes of neurones and glia of rat brain. *Biokhimiya*, **38**, 298–303.

Rees, D. & Usherwood, P. N. R. (1972). Fine structure of normal and degenerating motor axons and nerve-muscle synapses in the locust, *Schistocerca gregaria*. Comparative Biochemistry and Physiology, **43A**, 83–101.

Repke, H. & Maderspach, K. (1982). Muscarinic acetylcholine receptors on cultured glia cells. *Brain Research*, **232**, 206–11.

Rind, F. C. (1984). A chemical synapse between two motion detecting neurones in the locust brain. *Journal of Experimental Biology*, **110**, 143–67.

Roberts, A. M., Krasne, F. B., Hagiwara, G., Wine, J. J. & Kramer, A. P. (1982). Segmental giant: evidence for a driver neuron interposed between command and motor neurones in the crayfish escape system. *Journal of Neurophysiology*, **47**, 761–81.

Robinson, G. A., Butcher, R. W. & Sutherland, E. W. (1971). *Cyclic AMP*. Academic Press, New York.

Roper, S. (1976). An electrophysiological study of chemical and electrical synapses on neurones in the parasympathetic cardiac ganglion of the mudpuppy *Necturus maculosis*: evidence for intrinsic ganglionic innervation. *Journal of Physiology*, **254**, 427–54.

Ross, E. M. & Gilman, A. G. (1977). Resolution of some components of adenylate cyclase necessary for catalytic activity. *Journal of Biological Chemistry*, **252**, 6966–9.

Ross, E. M., Howlett, A. C., Ferguson, K. M. & Gilman, A. G. (1978). Reconstruction of hormone-sensitive adenylate cyclase activity with resolved components of the enzyme. *Journal of Biological Chemistry*, **253**, 6401–12.

Roth, J. (1982). The preparation of protein A-gold complexes with 3 nm and 15 nm gold particles and their use in labelling multiple antigens on ultra-thin sections. *Histochemical Journal*, **14**, 791–801.

Ruda, M. A. & Coulter, J. D. (1982). Axonal transport and trans-neuronal transport of wheatgerm agglutinin demonstrated by im-munocytochemistry. *Brain Research*, **249**, 237–46.

Sanders-Bush, E. (1987). 5HT receptors: Transmembrane signaling mechanisms in neuronal sertonin. eds. N. N. Osborne & M. Hamon. Wiley, Chichester, pp. 449–64.

Schächter, M., Godfrey, P. P., Minchin, M. C. W., McClue, S. J. & Young, M. M. (1984). Serotonin agonists stimulate inositol lipid meta-bolism in rabbit platelets. *Life Sciences*, **37**, 1641–7.

Schlichter, D. J., Casnellie, J. E. & Greengard, P. (1978). An endoge-nous substrate for cGMP-dependent protein kinase in mammalian cerebellum. *Nature*, **273**, 61–2.

Schönitzer, K. & Holländer, H. (1981). Anterograde tracing of horseradish peroxidase (HRP) with the electron microscope using the tetramethyl benzidine reaction. *Journal of Neuroscience Methods*, **4**, 373–83.

Schubert, D., Tarikas, H. & La Corbiere, M. (1976). Neuotransmitter regulation of adenosine-3′,5′-monophosphate in clonal nerve, glia and muscle cell lines. *Science*, 192, 471–2.

Schwab, M. E. & Thoenen, H. (1976). Electron microscopic evidence for a trans-synaptic migration of tetanus toxin in spinal cord motoneurones: an autoradiographic and morphometric study. *Brain Research*, 105, 213–27.

Schwab, M., Agid, Y., Glowinski, J. & Thoenen, H. (1977). Retrograde transport of 125-I-tetanus toxin as a tool for tracing fibre connections in the central nervous system: connections of the rostral part of the rat neo-striatum. *Brain Research*, 126, 211–24.

Schwab, M. E., Javoy-Agid, F. & Agid, Y. (1978). Labelled wheatgerm agglutinin (WGA) as a new, highly sensitive retrograde tracer in the rat brain hippocampal system. *Brain Research*, 152, 145–50.

Schwartz, J. P. & Costa, E. (1977). Regulation of nerve growth factor content in C6 glioma cells by β-adrenergic receptor stimulation. *Archives of Pharmacology*, 300, 123–9.

Seal, L. H. & Pentreath, V. W. (1985). Modulation of glial glycogen metabolism by 5-hydroxytryptamine in leech segmental ganglia. *Neurochemistry International*, 7, 1037–45.

Sellinger, O. Z., Azcurra, J. M., Johnoson, D. E., Ohesson, W. G. & Londin, Z. (1971). Independence of protein synthesis and drug uptake in nerve cell bodies and glial cells isolated by a new technique. *Nature*, 230, 253–6.

Shimihara, T. & Tauc, L. (1975). Multiple interneuronal afferents to the giant cells in *Aplysia*. *Journal of Physiology*, 247, 299–319.

Simpson, I., Rose, B. & Loewenstein, W. R. (1977). Size limit of molecules permeating the junctional membrane channels. *Science*, 195, 294–6.

Sjostrand, F. S. (1953). Ultrastructure of retinal rod synapses of guinea-pig eye. *Journal Applied Physics*, 24, 1422–3.

Snow, P. J., Rose, P. K. & Brown, A. G. (1976). Tracing axons and axon collaterals of spinal neurones using intracellular injection of horseradish peroxidase. *Science*, 191, 312–3.

Sokoloff, L. (1977). Relation between histological function and energy metabolism in the central nervous system. *Journal of Neurochemistry*, 29, 13–26.

Somogyi, P. (1978). The study of Golgi stained cells and of experimental degeneration under the electron microscope: a direct method for the identification in the visual cortex of three successive links in a neuron chain. *Neuroscience*, 3, 167–80.

Somogyi, P. & Smith, A. D. (1979). Projection of neostriatal spiny neurons to the substantia nigra. Application of a combined Golgi-staining and horseradish peroxidase transport procedure at both light and electron microscopic levels. *Brain Research*, **178**, 3–15.

Somogyi, P. & Soltés, I. (1986). Immuno-gold demonstration of GABA in synaptic terminals of intracellularly recorded horse-radish peroxidase-filled basket cells and clutch cells in the cat's visual cortex. *Neuroscience*, **19**, 1051–65.

Sotelo, C. & Palay, S. (1968). The fine structure of the lateral vestibular nucleus in the rat. I. Neurons and neuroglia. *Journal of Cell Biology*, **36**, 151–79.

Spray, D. C. & Bennett, M. V. L. (1985). Physiology and pharmacology of gap junctions. *Annual Review of Physiology*, **47**, 281–303.

Spray, D. C., Harris, A. L. & Bennett, M. V. L. (1979). Voltage dependence of junctional conductance in early amphibian embryos. *Science*, **204**, 432–4.

Spray, D. C., White, R. L., Verselis, V. & Bennett, M. V. L. (1985). General and comparative physiology of gap junction channels. In: *Gap Junctions*, eds. M. V. L. Bennett & D. C. Spray, pp. 139–53. Cold Spring Harbor Laboratory.

Staun-Olsen, P. P, Ottesen, B., Bartels, P. D., Nielsen, M. H., Gammeltoft, S. & Fahrenkrug, J. (1982). Receptors for vasoactive intestinal polypeptide in isolated synaptosomes from rat cerebral cortex. Heterogeneity of binding and desensitisation of receptors. *Journal of Neurochemistry*, **39**, 1242–51.

Sternberger, L. A. (1979). *Immunocytochemistry*. John Wiley & Sons, New York.

Sternberger, L. A., Hardy, P. H., Cuculis, J. J. & Meyer, H. G. (1970). The unlabelled antibody–enzyme method of immunohistochemistry. Preparation and properties of soluble antigen-antibody complex (horseradish peroxidase antiHorseradish-peroxidase) and its use in the identification of spirochetes. *Journal of Histochemistry and Cytochemistry*, **18**, 315–33.

Stewart, W. W. (1981). Lucifer dyes – highly fluorescent dyes for biological tracing. *Nature*, **292**, 17–21.

Stirling, C. A. (1972). The ultrastructure of giant fibre and serial synapses in crayfish. *Zeitschrift für Zellforschung and mikroskopsiche Anatomie*, **131**, 31–45.

Stoeckel, K., Schwab, N. & Thoenen, H. (1975). Specificity of retrograde transport of nerve growth factor (NGF) in sensory neurons: A biochemical and morphological study. *Brain Research*, **89**, 1–14.

Streb, H., Irvine, R. F., Berridge, M. J. & Schulz, I. (1983). Release of Ca^{2+} from a non-mitochondrial intracellular store in pancreatic acina cells by inositol-1,4,5-triphosphate. *Nature*, 306, 67–9.

Streit, P. (1980). Selective retrograde labelling indicating the transmitter of neuronal pathways. *Journal of Comparative Neurology*, **191**, 429–63.

Streit, P., Knecht, E., Reubi, J-C., Hunt, S. P. & Cuénod, M. (1978). GABA-specific presynaptic dendrites in pigeon optic tectum: a high resolution autoradiographic study. *Brain Research*, **149**, 204–10.

Strumwasser, F. (1962). Postsynaptic inhibition and excitation produced by different branches of a single neuron and the common transmitter involved. *International Congress of Physiological Science*, **22**, No. 801.

Suguria, Y., Lee, C. L. & Perl, E. R. (1986). Central projections of functionally identified, unmyelinated (C) afferent fibres in mammalian cutaneous nerve. *Science*, **234**, 358–61.

Sulser, F. (1979). New perspectives on the mode of action of antidepressant drugs. *Trends in Pharmacological Sciences*, **1**, 92–6.

Tanouye, M. A. & Wyman, R. J. (1980). Motor outputs of giant nerve fiber in *Drosophila*. *Journal of Neurophysiology*, **45**, 405–21.

Trauc, L. L. (1977). Transmitter release at cholinergic synapses. In *Synapses*, eds. Cottrell, G. A. and Usherwood, P. N. R., pp. 64–78. Blackie, Glasgow.

Tobin, A. B. & Osborne, N. N. (1988). Evidence for the presence of serotonin nerves and receptors in the iris–ciliary body complex of the rabbit. *Journal of Neuroscience*, **8**, 3713–21.

Triller, A., Cluzeaud, F., Pfeiffer, F., Betz, H. & Korn, H. (1985). Distribution of glycine receptors at central synapses: an immunoelectron microscopical study. *Journal of Cell Biology*, **101**, 683–8.

Trimble, W. S. & Scheller, R. H. (1988). Molecular biology of synaptic vesicle associated proteins. *Trends in Neuroscience*, **11**, 241–2.

Trojanowski, J. Q. & Schmidt, M. L. (1984). Interneuronal transfer of axonally transported proteins: studies with HRP and HRP conjugates of wheatgerm agglutinin, cholera toxin and the B subunit of cholera toxin. *Brain Research*, **311**, 366–9.

Trojanowski, J. Q., Gonatas, J. O. & Gonatas, N. K. (1981). Conjugates of horseradish peroxidase (HRP) with cholera toxin and wheatgerm agglutinin are superior to free HRP as orthogradely transported markers. *Brain Research*, **223**, 381–5.

Tweedle, C. D. (1978). Single-cell staining techniques: In: *Neuroanatomical research techniques*, ed. R. T. Robertson. Academic Press, New York.

Unwin, P. N. T. & Zampighi, G. (1980). Structure of the gap junction between communicating cells. *Nature (London)*, **283**, 545–9.

Usherwood, P. N. R. & Rees, D. (1972). Quantitative studies of spatial distribution of synaptic vesicles within normal and degenerating axons of the locust, *Schistocerca gregaria*. *Comparative Biochemistry and Physiology*, **43A**, 103–18.

Van Calker, D., Muller, M. & Hamprecht, B. (1978). Adrenergic alpha- and beta-receptors expressed by the same cell type in primary culture of perinatal mouse brain. *Journal of Neurochemistry*, **30**, 713–18.

Van Calker, D., Muller, M. & Hamprecht, B. (1979). Receptors regulating the level of cyclic AMP in primary cultures of perinatal mouse brain. In: *Neural Growth and Differentiation*, eds. E. Meisami & M. A. B. Brazier, pp. 11–25. Raven Press, New York.

van der Kooy, D., Kuypers, H. G. J. M. & Catsman-Berrevoets, C. E. (1978). Single mamillary body cells with divergent axon collaterals. Demonstration by a simple fluorescent retrograde double labelling technique in the rat. *Brain Research*, **158**, 189–96.

Verselis, V., White, R. L., Spray, D. C. & Bennett, M. V. L. (1986). Gap junctional conductance and permeability are linearly related. *Science*, **234**, 461–4.

Von Hungen, K., Roberts, S., & Hill, D. F. (1974). Development and regional variations in neurotransmitter-sensitive adenylate cyclase system in cell-free preparations from the rat brain. *Journal of Neurochemistry*, **22**, 811–19.

Walberg, F. (1964). The early changes in degenerating boutons and the problem of argyrophilia. *Journal of Comparative Neurology*, **187**, 113–37.

Wan, X.S.T., Trojanowski, J. Q., Gonatas, J. O. & Liu, C. N. (1982). Cytoarchitecture of the extranuclear and commisural dendrites of hypoglossal nucleus as revealed by conjugates of horseradish peroxidase with cholera toxin. *Experimental Neurology*, **78**, 167–75.

Watson, S. P. (1984). The action of substance P on contraction inositol phospholipid and adenylate cyclase in rat small intestine. *Biochemical Pharmacology*, **33**, 3733–7.

Westfall, D. P., Stitzel, R. E. & Rowe, J. N. (1978). The postjunctional effects and neuronal release of purine compounds in guinea-pig vas deferens. *European Journal of Pharmacology*, **50**, 27–38.

Wharton, J., Polak, J. M., Probert, L., De Mey, J., McGregor, G. P., Bryant, M. G. & Bloom, S. R. (1981). Peptide containing nerves in the ureter of the guineapig and cat. *Neuroscience*, **6**, 969–82.

Whittaker, V. P. (1966). Some properties of synaptic membranes isolated from the central nervous system. *Annals of the New York Academy of Science*, **137**, 982–98.

Wine, J. J. (1977). Neuronal organization of crayfish escape behavior: inhibition of the giant motoneuron via a disynaptic pathway from other motoneurons. *Journal of Neurophysiology*, **40**, 1078–97.

Winlow, W. and Benjamin, P. R. (1977). Postsynaptic effects of a multi-action giant interneurone on identified snail neurones. *Nature*, **268**, 263–5.

Winlow, W., Haydon, P. G. & Benjamin, P. R. (1981). Multiple postsynaptic actions of the giant dopamine-containing neurone R. Pe. D. 1 of *Lymnaea stagnalis* (L). *Journal of Experimental Biology*, **4**, 137–48.

Winlow, W. & Usherwood, P. N. R. (1975). Ultrastructural studies of normal and degenerating mouse neuromuscular junctions. *Journal of Neurocytology*, **4**, 377–94.

Winlow, W. & Usherwood, P. N. R. (1976). Electrophysiological studies of normal and degenerating mouse neuromuscular junctions. *Brain Research*, **110**, 447–61.

Wouterlood, F. G. & Mugnani, E. (1984). Cartwheel neurones of the dorsal cochlear nucleus: a Golgi-electron microscopic study in the rat. *Journal of Comparative Neurology*, **227**, 136–57.

Wouterlood, F. G. & Groenwegen, H. J. (1985). Neuroanatomical tracing by use of *Phaseolus vulgaris-leucoagglutinin (PHA-L): electron microscopy of PHA-L filled somata, dendrites, axons and axon terminals*. *Brain Research*, **326**, 188–91.

Yasargil, G. M. and Diamond, J. (1968). Startle response in teleost fish: an elementary circuit for neural discrimination. *Nature*, **220**, 241–3.

Yousufzai, S. Y. K., Akhtar, R. A. & Abdel-Latif, A. A. (1986). Effects of substance P on inositol triphosphate accumulation on contractile responses and on arachidonic acid release and prostaglandin biosynthesis in rabbit iris sphincter muscle. *Experiental Eye Research*, **43**, 215–26.

Index